100 Questions & Answers About Mesothelioma

THIRD EDITION

Harvey I. Pass, MD

Stephen E. Banner Professor of Thoracic Oncology
Vice Chair, Research, Department of Cardiothoracic Surgery
Director, Division of Thoracic Surgery and Thoracic Oncology
Department of Cardiothoracic Surgery
NYU Langone Medical Center and School of Medicine
New York, NY

Mary Hesdorffer, NP

Executive Director
Mesothelioma Applied Research Foundation
(Meso Foundation)
Alexandria, VA

Sarah Elizabeth Lake

Sarah Ann Lake

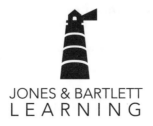

JONES & BARTLETT
LEARNING

World Headquarters
Jones & Bartlett Learning
5 Wall Street
Burlington, MA 01803
978-443-5000
info@jblearning.com
www.jblearning.com

Jones & Bartlett Learning books and products are available through most bookstores and online booksellers. To contact Jones & Bartlett Learning directly, call 800-832-0034, fax 978-443-8000, or visit our website, www.jblearning.com.

Substantial discounts on bulk quantities of Jones & Bartlett Learning publications are available to corporations, professional associations, and other qualified organizations. For details and specific discount information, contact the special sales department at Jones & Bartlett Learning via the above contact information or send an email to specialsales@jblearning.com.

Production Credits

Executive Publisher: Christopher Davis
Managing Editor: Kathy Richardson
Production Editor: Daniel Stone
Manufacturing and Inventory Control Supervisor: Amy Bacus
Editorial Assistant: Marisa LaFleur
Marketing: Jean O'Neil

Composition: Jason Miranda, Spoke & Wheel
Cover Images: Top Left: © Gorgev/ShutterStock, Inc.; Top Right: © Ryan McVay/Lifesize/ Thinkstock; Bottom: © iStockphoto/Thinkstock
Printing and Binding: Edwards Brothers Malloy
Cover Printing: Edwards Brothers Malloy

Library of Congress Cataloging-in-Publication Data
100 questions and answers about mesothelioma / Harvey I. Pass ... [et al.]. — 3rd ed.
   p. cm.
  Rev. ed. of: 100 questions & answers about mesothelioma / Harvey I. Pass, Amy Metula, Susan Vento. 2nd ed. c2010.
  Includes index.
  ISBN 978-1-4496-8808-0 (alk. paper)
1. Mesothelioma—Popular works. 2. Mesothelioma—Miscellanea. I. Pass, Harvey I. II. 100 questions & answers about mesothelioma. III. Title: One hundred questions and answers about mesothelioma.
  RC280.L8P375 2013
  616.99'42—dc23
                              2012024205
6048

Printed in the United States of America
18 17   10

CONTENTS

So here we are again with another edition of a book that I wish you never had to get and I didn't have to do another version. I have been trying to figure out this disease for 25 years now, either in the lab, in the operating room, listening to my contemporaries at meetings or at tumor boards, and it is safe to say that I remain humbled and frustrated. I can't tell patients for certain whether they are going to respond to therapy; I can't tell patients I have the magic biomarker that can detect the disease at an early stage where the chance for a cure is much higher; I can't tell patients how long they are going to live or whether their tumor is aggressive or not. I can only advise patients what my experience has been over this 25-year period and tell them the truth: mesothelioma is a tough disease to deal with from the patient's and family's standpoint as well as from the treating physician's standpoint, BUT we have made progress. I give you my word that 25 years ago there weren't as many oncologists who knew about the disease; there weren't surgeons all over the United States who had been trained to perform the surgical procedures by experts in New York, Boston, or Houston; and there were no combination therapies that had a response rate consistently greater than 10%. What's the best situation now for patients and families with mesothelioma? They have more choices! We are not fixated on only one surgical procedure, and the risk for surgery at specialized centers is five fold less than it was when I was training. There are more systemic chemotherapies that can be delivered safely and have a greater chance of shrinking the tumors. There are resources like the Meso Foundation that are actually helping to guide patients and their families through this part of their lives where they try desparately to maintain control of life when life seems to be out of control. This book is meant to be a resource, too. You need information and you need to be forearmed when you meet people who you hoped you would never have to see.

This book in no way answers every question ... how could it? We only discuss 100 of them. However, it's a start, and I am convinced that the knowledge about this disease is accelerating on all fronts: clinical trials, the laboratory, personalizing surgery, and early detection.

And, after all, for the rest of the questions you know where to reach us, and we are there for you.

Harvey I. Pass, MD

I began work with mesothelioma patients 2 years into my career never realizing that it would become my life's work and passion. In my role as a nurse and then nurse practitioner I have had the opportunity to become directly involved with hundreds of mesothelioma patients and their family members. My interest in assisting Dr. Pass with this book is that I believe that you as a patient or family member, once educated about the disease, can be successful in managing mesothelioma and all the changes it brings to your life and that of your loved ones. Initially the diagnosis creates chaos and a loss of control. This book was written to give you back that control and to assist you in gaining necessary knowledge to partner with your healthcare team to design a comprehensive treatment plan and live the best life possible despite the diagnosis of mesothelioma. The Mesothelioma Applied Research Foundation (the Meso Foundation) is here to continue updating you on disease advancements, provide supportive counseling, either in group or individualized format, to help you to identify promising clinical trials, and finally to partner with you to fund the necessary research to find a cure.

Mary Hesdorffer, NP

For our family March 24, 2000, is one of those days you remember where you were and what you were doing. It was the day that our journey with mesothelioma would begin and a journey that would take us through almost 10 years of multiple surgeries, chemotherapy and radiation treatments, hip replacements, congestive heart failure, renal failure, and Phil would be placed on life support several times. There would be many struggles and hard times during those years, but it would also bring our family closer together and create a bond between us that would be strong enough to get us through mesothelioma and give Sarah Ann and myself the courage we would need to continue on with our lives without Phil.

Phil fought for every one of those days. He loved life and his family. He was willing to do just about anything for me and for our daughter who was only 10 years old at the time of his diagnosis. Phil set a goal to live long enough to see her graduate from high school. He lived to see that goal fulfilled and to even see her enter college and start out on her own journey in life.

Phil spoke at a Meso Foundation symposium one year about "Hope". Hope that mesothelioma would one day be eradicated. Hope that one day newly diagnosed patients and their families didn't have to hear the same words we heard—to go home and get your affairs in order. To prepare to die, soon. Hope that researchers were getting closer to a cure.

Our family felt truly blessed to have had great doctors. These doctors not only treated the cancer but were there for us also as fellow human beings. We were never just a number or another statistic to them. We believe that because of their expertise in each of their fields they were able to diagnose Phil quickly and get him the care he needed in a timely manner and give him the best chance at living a longer life. We truly appreciate and respect Dr. Harvey Pass, Dr. Robert Crisalli, and Dr. James Fram for their tireless efforts for Phil over the years. We were also fortunate to have an attorney, Stephen Johnston, who was able to assist us with asbestos litigation.

The one thing that mesothelioma did not take from our family was the determination we all shared. We would not allow it to take away our love and commitment we had for each other. We learned to lean on each other and make the most out of each day, to make as many good memories as possible to help us in the trying days that would lay ahead. We had support from both our parents and family members that were always just a phone call away. Phil and I met a couple while in the hospital recovering from his EPP, Mr. & Mrs. Jerry Krussell. A wonderful couple that we became very close to. Jerry also had mesothelioma and we were able to help one another through some difficult days. Jerry passed away several years after his surgery. Virginia and I remain close to this day and help support each other.

Lastly, it is our desire to see a cure for mesothelioma so that other families will not have to endure this disease. To see more funding for research so that doctors working tirelessly to help patients and their families will one day be able to look at a newly diagnosed patient and say there is Hope.

Sarah Lake and Sarah Ann Lake

We would like to acknowledge that many wonderful people that we have treated or come to know with this disease have actually contributed to making the lives of others a little better because they, both the patients and the families, have made us smarter about mesothelioma. There isn't a day that goes by that the editors don't think about these individuals, and that is part of *their* legacy.

The editors would also like to thank Bob Komitor for his insights about the legal aspects of mesothelioma.

PART ONE

The Basics

What is mesothelioma, and where does it come from?

What are the risk factors, or who gets mesothelioma?

Can mesothelioma be prevented?

More...

Pleural mesothelioma

Mesothelioma that originates in the chest cavity.

Pleural space

The space enclosed by the pleura, which is a thin layer of tissue that covers the lungs and lines the interior wall of the chest cavity.

Thoracic

Having to do with the chest.

Peritoneal mesothelioma

Mesothelioma that originates in the abdomen and/or pelvis.

Pericardium

The heart sac that covers the heart.

Pathologist

A doctor who identifies diseases by studying cells and tissues under a microscope.

Epithelial

Refers to the cells that line the internal and external surfaces of the body. Epithelial is also the term used to describe the appearance of the cells under the microscope for the most common type of mesothelioma.

1. What is mesothelioma?

Malignant mesothelioma, a rare form of cancer, originates in many of the protective linings that cover major organs in the abdomen and chest. There are approximately 3,500 people diagnosed each year in the United States. **Pleural mesothelioma**, the most common type of mesothelioma grows in the **pleural space** (the area between the chest wall and lung) and then progresses to the lung itself and other areas in the **thoracic** (chest) cavity. When it occurs in the abdomen, it is referred to as **peritoneal mesothelioma** and approximately 300 patients are diagnosed with this yearly in the United States. Other rare sites of occurrence include the **pericardium** (lining of the heart) and tunica vaginalis (lining membrane of the testicles), or scrotal lining.

2. Are there different types of mesothelioma?

Looking under the microscope, the **pathologist** is able to distinguish three distinct types of mesothelioma based on the appearance of the cells. The majority of mesothelioma is of the **epithelial** type, which, under the microscope, resembles adenocarcinoma cells (like those found in lung cancer). Special staining will be applied to your **biopsy** specimen to differentiate epithelial mesothelioma from **lung cancer** and from other tumors that are adenocarcinoma. **Sarcomatoid mesothelioma** is a more aggressive type of mesothelioma. Sarcomatoid occurs in approximately 7–20% of all malignant mesotheliomas. **Biphasic** or **mixed**, mesothelioma accounts for approximately 20–30% of malignant mesothelioma diagnoses, and is a combination of both epithelial and sarcomatoid mesothelioma.

As the field of mesothelioma science evolves, it is important to know the type of mesothelioma as we are developing agents that target **mesothelin**, a **protein** found on the outside of epithelial mesothelioma cells. This may prove to be a very important way of treating malignant mesothelioma by using "smart drugs" with known targets rather than a more generalized approach to treatment.

Surgical series are also reporting statistical differences among the various subtypes of mesothelioma. There are currently plans underway to develop strategies to determine who benefits from each type of treatment modality. In the future, we hope to guide the therapy for mesothelioma based on patients' unique cancer signature of proteins, genes, or other molecules.

3. What are the pleura?

In pleural mesothelioma the initial site of disease is most often the **pleura**, an important thin membrane that lines the inside of the chest wall (**parietal pleura**), or the **visceral pleura**, which lines the lungs. The pleura is a sheet-like lining formed by rectangular cells called **mesothelial cells**, and is usually not more than a few layers thick. If unaffected by disease, it is comparable in thickness to that of a blown-up balloon membrane. There are two pleuras in the chest. The parietal pleura lines the inside of the chest wall like wallpaper, covering not only the inside of the ribs but also the **diaphragm** and pericardium. The normal parietal pleura is no more than 2 to 3 mm thick, whereas the normal visceral pleura is fused to the lung and is about 1 mm thick. The visceral pleura is a separate pleura that covers the lung and is much more difficult to remove without

Biopsy
The removal of cells or tissues for examination under a microscope. When only a sample of tissue is removed, the procedure is called an incisional biopsy or core biopsy. When an entire lump or suspicious area is removed, the procedure is called an excisional biopsy. When a sample of tissue or fluid is removed with a needle, the procedure is called a needle biopsy or fine-needle aspiration. Pleural biopsies are used to make the diagnosis of mesothelioma.

Lung cancer
A cancer of the lungs that is comprised of different cells than those associated with mesothelioma.

Sarcomatoid mesothelioma
The least common variant of mesothelioma, which has the appearance under the microscope of spindly cells that look like supportive or connective tissue.

Biphasic
A mesothelioma that has both epithelial and sarcomatoid elements. Also called a mixed mesothelioma.

Mixed

A description of cells found in a mesothelioma tumor sample. Mixed histology, also referred to as biphasic, contains both sarcomatoid and epithelial cells and accounts for approximately 20–35% of mesotheliomas.

Mesothelin

A protein found on the outside of both normal and malignant cells. It is found in abundance in epithelial mesothelioma in addition to some other cancers.

Protein

A molecule made up of amino acids that are needed for the body to function properly.

Pleura

A thin layer of tissue covering the lungs and lining the interior wall of the chest cavity that protects and cushions the lungs.

Parietal pleura

The lining on the inside of the chest wall that is composed of mesothelial cells and is the target organ for asbestos-induced mesothelioma.

harming the lung. The job of the pleura is to filter fluid back and forth from the chest to the circulation. If the pleura become diseased, it is not as effective in eliminating fluid from the chest, and fluid accumulation (**pleural effusion**) can occur. You may be familiar with pleurisy, a nonmalignant condition whereby fluid accumulates in this space.

4. What are the risk factors, or who gets mesothelioma?

Anyone can get mesothelioma; it occurs across all races and genders and is found in young and old alike. The dominating risk factor in developing mesothelioma is exposure to **asbestos**. The risk is greatly increased in people who have had repeated exposure to asbestos for prolonged periods of time. The majority of people who develop this disease can trace their exposure back to jobs where they encountered asbestos. Thirty percent of all mesothelioma patients are navy veterans having been exposed in the boiler room of the ships or working in the shipyards. Other high-risk professions include brake repair workers, construction workers, those who worked with or manufactured insulation materials, and people who work in asbestos abatement (removal of asbestos).

We often talk of "secondhand" exposure, which would affect those who came into contact with mesothelioma through asbestos fibers brought home on workers' clothing and equipment. Many people are exposed at home, schools, or office buildings during renovation projects.

It has been reported that the **Simian virus 40 (SV40)**, a virus that contaminated the polio vaccine between 1954 and 1963, may increase the risk of developing mesothelioma in asbestos-exposed individuals who harbor this virus. This virus was first found in rhesus monkeys and is now found in the human population. Though the vaccine no longer contains the virus, an unknown proportion of the population is infected with the virus despite not having received a contaminated strain of the vaccine. It is thought that it may be spread through human feces, breast milk, and semen. The virus alone has not demonstrated the ability to cause mesothelioma but one hypothesis is that it can act along with asbestos to increase the risk of mesothelioma in humans. This has been demonstrated in cell and animal **tissue** experiments. The relevance of this finding is still under investigation.

Patients who previously received high doses of **radiation** therapy for prior malignancies can develop mesothelioma and other more common cancers. Usually patients have been treated for lymphoma in the chest. Nevertheless, there are very few reports in the medical literature of mesothelioma developing after radiation therapy and with asbestos being so widely used and so many people unknowingly exposed, it is difficult to tell whether these people were also exposed to asbestos at some time in their lives.

Lastly, there are data that a person's own **genes** can play an important role in determining who is susceptible to these mineral fibers and will then develop mesothelioma. Recently a genetic mutation has been found that makes an individual more susceptible to mesothelioma and melanoma of the eye. Hopefully this finding will benefit patients suffering from these diseases not only for the development of new treatment options, but also in developing early detection strategies in high-risk individuals who carry this mutation and who are exposed to

Visceral pleura

The mesothelial lining on the surface of the lung that can also be a target organ for mesothelioma.

Mesothelial cells

A specialized layer of cells that form a thin layer along the cavity and internal organs. These cells are responsible for secretions that aid in cellular processes.

Diaphragm

The major muscle separating the abdomen from the chest.

Pleural effusion

An abnormal collection of fluid between the thin layers of tissue lining the lung and the wall of the chest cavity (pleura).

Asbestos

A naturally occurring mineral composed of long thin fibers which, when inhaled or swallowed, are directly implicated in the development of mesothelioma, asbestosis, lung cancer, and medical conditions.

THE BASICS

asbestos. It is anticipated that more genes with similar properties will be discovered in studies that will uncover all the known mutations in mesothelioma.

Sarah adds...

It was unbelievable to learn that asbestos surrounds all of us. It can be found in our schools, work places, and our homes. The fact that we can do something as simple as going to school or work and that could put us in harm's way is difficult to think about.

5. What causes mesothelioma?

We know that exposure to asbestos causes mesothelioma. This has been proven in the research laboratory, as well as in animal experiments and in studies of exposed human beings. Recently researchers at Mt. Sinai Hospital in New York City reviewed the autopsies of 2,015 patients who died between 1883 and 1910. This review did not reveal any cases of tumors that resembled mesothelioma, apparently due to the fact that asbestos was not in generalized use during this period of time. This adds to the mounting evidence that asbestos is a key factor in the development of this disease.

We have no evidence regarding the necessary level of asbestos for an individual to be exposed to in order to develop a mesothelioma. We only know that people who end up with this disease usually have had some type of previous exposure to asbestos. When asbestos is inhaled, it can travel and eventually lodge itself in tissue. It is thought that this leads to inflammation and or irritation. It is not fully understood if asbestos fibers themselves cause the cells to release cytokines (body chemicals that induce cells to become cancerous) or if the tissues when injured lead to the release of chemicals (cytokines) that direct the cells to become malignant. It is hypothesized that asbestos fibers are inhaled and first travel through the upper air passages, which include the throat, trachea (windpipe), and large bronchi (large breathing tubes of the lungs). Normally if an irritant is detected, we have a cough reflex to clear secretions and foreign bodies. Asbestos fibers are long and thin and may not be detected by the system we rely on to protect the lungs from foreign material. Once asbestos fibers are imbedded in the pleura, they can cause injury, which leads to the development of **pleural plaques** (calcium containing plate-like structures) or **fibrosis** (scar tissue). When the lung itself is injured, these damaged areas create scar tissue known as **asbestosis**. Asbestosis can be associated with lung cancer or mesothelioma, though patients with pleural plaques are thought to be at the highest risk for developing mesothelioma. In peritoneal mesothelioma, it is thought that these fibers travel via the **lymph** or blood stream, or are simply swallowed and end up in the abdomen. It is difficult to find these fibers when examining the tissues of the abdomen but oftentimes we see peritoneal patients with pleural plaques, which is irrefutable evidence of asbestos exposure.

6. Can mesothelioma be prevented?

Avoiding exposure to asbestos is the best way to prevent the development of mesothelioma. The **Occupational Safety and Health Administration (OSHA)** is the federal agency responsible for developing safety regulations for workers who come into contact with asbestos. Employers are required to follow these regulations and to ensure that their workers have adequate education about safety and the use of protective equipment.

THE BASICS

Fibrosis

The growth of tissue containing or resembling fibers that can occur after radiation therapy or as scarring after any disruption of normal tissue.

Asbestosis

A lung disease caused by exposure to asbestos. The lungs lose their natural elasticity, resulting in difficulty moving air into and out of the lungs.

Lymph

Fluid composed of lymphocytes.

Occupational Safety and Health Administration (OSHA)

A government agency that regulates the use of asbestos and sets the standards for its distribution.

Secondhand exposure

Exposure to asbestos that occurs indirectly, such as from someone else's clothing, as opposed to exposure in the working place.

Environmental Protection Agency (EPA)

The mission of the EPA is to protect human health and the environment.

Amphibole

A type of asbestos also known as brown or blue asbestos named for company that began mining it in South African. Exposure to this form of asbestos is known to cause mesothelioma, lung cancer, and other medical conditions.

3,000 products containing asbestos were in general use up until the late 1980s.

Serpentine

A type of asbestos known as white or blue asbestos. The majority (95%) of the asbestos found in the United States is of this type.

Workers should bring any concerns regarding the safe handling of asbestos to both their employees and union representatives. Workers should also be aware of the risk of bringing home asbestos fibers on their work clothes, skin, hair, and tools. Proper handling of contaminated items should be implemented. Showering at work and changing out of work clothes prior to entering the home can greatly lower the chance of **secondhand exposure**.

If you are considering doing home repair or remodeling, you should be aware that approximately 3,000 products containing asbestos were in general use up until the late 1980s. You need to use caution when attempting any type of home repair and should consult with experts if you suspect asbestos. The **Environmental Protection Agency (EPA)** has a comprehensive booklet that describes asbestos in the home. If you are aware of asbestos in your home or workplace, contact a reputable asbestos abatement company to guarantee safe removal of affected areas. Do not attempt to remove asbestos on your own; hire trained professionals and check their credentials before initiating the work.

Did you know that asbestos is also a causative agent in many cases of lung cancer? Many studies have reported that people who smoke and have asbestos exposure have a sevenfold increase over smokers with no asbestos exposure in the development of lung cancer. Unlike lung cancer, mesothelioma is not caused by cigarettes unless the smoker was also exposed to asbestos.

If you are a smoker, quit now and tell other individuals you know who have been exposed to asbestos to quit smoking.

7. What is asbestos?

Asbestos is the term used for a naturally occurring mineral that resembles a rock in its natural form. The rock is then split into fibers, which are resistant to heat, fire, and chemicals. These natural properties made it a popular commercial product used indiscriminately in the United States until the late 1970s. The fibers once woven into fine thread can become brittle and can then float in the air, where they can be inhaled, land on and stick to clothing, and found on exposed surfaces of a person's body who has been exposed to these fibers.

Asbestos fibers are divided into two distinct groups: **amphibole** and **serpentine**. Amphibole, which has long needle-like threads, is more brittle than serpentine and is more limited in its ability to be fabricated. Both of these groups are associated with mesothelioma, lung cancer, asbestosis, and other malignancies.

Recently other types of minerals have been found to be associated with asbestos, including **tremolite, taconite** and **erionite**. **Vermiculite** from the region of Libby, MT was contaminated with tremolite. Unfortunately, vermiculite from Libby has been used in insulation as well as soil for potting plants. Taconite, a mineral that is mined mostly in Minnesota, has also been associated with the development of mesothelioma. It is not known if taconite itself causes mesothelioma or if this association is because soil near taconite mines is frequently contaminated with asbestos. The concern has been the rising incidence of mesothelioma among taconite miners. Erinoite, another mineral found to cause mesothelioma in villages in Turkey, has been found in select locations in the United States, but so far no cases of mesothelioma in the United States have been directly traced to this mineral.

THE BASICS

Tremolite
A type of asbestos which has contaminated the vermiculite mined in Libby, MT, and also has contaminated chrysotile (a serpentine asbestos) and talc.

Taconite
A rock that contains approximately 25% iron and as iron stores in the United States diminished, this rock became prized for its ability to extract iron from within the rock. This mineral is heavily mined in Minnesota, where an association with higher-than-expected cases of mesothelioma and asbestos-related diseases has been reported.

Erionite
A naturally occurring mineral in the zeolite family of minerals with properties similar to asbestos.

Vermiculite
A naturally occurring mineral that is used for insulation. In Libby, MT, the vermiculite mine was contaminated with asbestos and many people have been exposed to asbestos and developed asbestos-related diseases due to this contamination.

PART TWO

Diagnosis

What are the symptoms of mesothelioma?

Should I get a second opinion?

How do I find the best doctors to
treat my mesothelioma?

More...

8. What are the symptoms of mesothelioma?

Mesothelioma symptoms can mimic those found in many other cancers as well as benign diseases. Diagnosing mesothelioma from symptoms is never accurate, so diagnosing requires very careful testing. Mesothelioma is often not suspected since it is so rare and many patients do not equate their asbestos exposure to their current medical complaints. The great majority of patients are diagnosed in their later years with the average age of **diagnosis** reported at 70 years of age. Following exposure to asbestos, malignant mesothelioma can develop 10–50 years later and though the majority of patients have had a work history with asbestos exposure, there is a significant number of patients who have had secondhand exposure (asbestos fibers brought home on clothing from a work place that or exposure through construction and remodeling). This secondhand exposure can result in patients being unaware that they might have been exposed to this deadly fiber, leaving a crucial gap in their medical history.

All patients are unique and not only do they have different symptoms but they also have unique ways of describing them. When the pleura is affected, patients may complain of a tightness in the chest, most likely due to the pleura beginning to lose its elasticity. They may complain of an inability to take a deep breath, possibly due to stiffness of the diaphragm from tumor or fluid, thus preventing the lungs from expanding fully. Persistent **cough** and **dyspnea** (shortness of breath) may be secondary to fluid that accumulates as a pleural effusion or around the heart (**pericardial effusion**). Difficulty swallowing and hoarseness is occasionally described. During the course of their illness, the vast majority of patients

Diagnosis

The process of identifying a disease by the signs and symptoms.

Cough

The mechanism by which we clear irritants from the large breathing passages.

Dyspnea

Difficult, painful breathing or shortness of breath; one of the early symptoms of mesothelioma in the pleura due to the accumulation of fluid in the chest.

Pericardial effusion

A collection of fluid in the space between the heart and the sac-like protective tissue, the pericardium.

will have to contend with a pleural effusion. Pain can develop early in the course of the disease and may be related to invasion into the muscle of the chest wall or rarely, mesothelioma will invade directly into ribs. Very often this pain is located over the lower portion of the chest and extending to the back and sides. There may also be pain at the biopsy site, sometimes associated with tumor seeding along the needle or biopsy track. Other symptoms of disease may include weight loss and night sweats. Basic laboratory studies, such as the complete blood count (CBC), may demonstrate an elevation of white cell or **platelet** counts. In some individuals, an **anemia** (low **red blood cell** count) may be noted, which is termed the anemia of chronic disease (or more correctly, the anemia of chronic inflammation).

In peritoneal mesothelioma, patients often complain of tightness and swelling of the abdomen. Weight loss varies as some patients will lose muscle mass, but patients will gain weight as fluid accumulates in the abdomen. Pain is most often experienced in patients with advanced disease due to invasion of soft tissue, such as muscle or bone. Night sweats are a common complaint as are the changes in blood counts described above.

Sarah adds . . .

Phil was working away from home in Wilmington, DE when he started to have what he thought was the flu. He felt tired, had a cough, and had noticed that he seemed to get short of breath very easily. He tried to treat these symptoms with over-the-counter medications, but realized after several weeks he wasn't improving and decided he needed to go to a medical facility for further evaluation. His initial concern and delay in seeking medical care was that he was going to miss a day of work by going to a doctor. By that evening he was in a hospital emergency room and they were draining

Platelet

A type of blood cell that helps prevent bleeding by causing blood clots to form; also called a thrombocyte.

Anemia

A condition in which the number of red blood cells is below normal.

Red blood cell

A cell that carries oxygen to all parts of the body; also called an erythrocyte.

1600 cc of bloody fluid by performing a thoracentesis. That day started what would become an almost 10-year battle with mesothelioma for our family.

9. How is mesothelioma diagnosed?

Doctors attempt to diagnose illnesses based upon the most common diseases that might account for those symptoms. Hence, if the doctor does not ask about exposure to fibers, he will not consider mesothelioma. Therefore, if you or your friends have worked with asbestos or have a known exposure, it is very important to make this part of your health record. A history of tobacco use is also important as patients who smoke and have asbestos exposure have a much higher incidence of lung cancer than smokers without asbestos exposure. If you have already been diagnosed with asbestosis or have pleural plaques (areas of scarring on the lung from asbestos), you should bring any changes in symptoms to the attention of your medical team rather than waiting for your next scheduled appointment as under those circumstances, your doctor will definitely consider a more thorough evaluation to make sure that you have not progressed on to develop a mesothelioma. Shortness of breath, pain, abdominal swelling, unexplained weight gain or loss, and any other unusual symptoms should prompt you to call your physician, stressing your exposure to asbestos and the need to compare prior chest X-ray findings with a new study. The initial consultation will be to record your symptoms and based on these symptoms, an individualized series of investigations will be initiated. You will be asked a series of questions or provided with a form to fill out asking about any changes noted since your last exam with specific regard to issues such as sleep patterns, changes in appetite, unintentional weight

Shortness of breath, pain, abdominal swelling, unexplained weight gain or loss, and any other unusual symptoms should prompt you to call your physician.

loss or gain, shortness of breath, chest pain and night sweats, chills, or fevers. If you are having any unusual symptoms, this is the time to bring them to the attention of your doctor.

Some patients feel nervous or uncomfortable at doctor's visits. There is an easy solution to this: In advance of your visit, prepare a list of questions for the doctor and list the changes you may have noted at home. Think about your family history, including the occupations of your parents, and jot down some notes about your family's cancer history as well as other major medical illnesses that may have affected your family members.

During the physical exam the physician will listen to your lungs and may note an absence or unusual breath sounds as he or she listens closely with the stethoscope. He or she will then correlate these changes to the symptoms that you discussed prior to the physical exam. You will undoubtedly be sent for a chest X-ray to determine if the cause of these changes will be evident on the film, and if there is a change from previous X-rays. If a mass or fluid is noted in the lung or an irregular shape is seen attached to your pleura, you will most likely be sent for additional X-rays and/or scans. If there is fluid, a sample may be collected by aspiration using a needle that penetrates the pleural space, and this fluid will be sent for further specific chemical testing as well as a microscopic examination. Blood work will also be performed to gather additional information about your health status and to help in the overall diagnostic process.

When the doctor examines your abdomen, he or she may note distention (swelling) or a change in bowel sounds, or may feel abnormal masses. You will most likely be sent for a **CT scan** and/or ultrasound and, if

CT scan

A series of detailed pictures of areas inside the body, taken from different angles; the pictures are created by a computer linked to an X-ray machine. Also called computerized axial tomography, computed tomography, or computerized tomography.

DIAGNOSIS

fluid is demonstrated, a needle aspiration to obtain a sample of that fluid, either by your doctor or the radiologist. If a mass is noted, along with other significant changes in one or more of these radiological studies, additional tests will be ordered and ultimately again, a biopsy will be performed. A radiologist will most likely perform this biopsy, but a surgeon will perform it if the mass to be biopsied is not easily within reach of a needle or is in a spot where complications could occur if only radiological guidance is used.

Peritoneum

The membrane the forms the lining of the abdominal cavity.

Prognosis

The likely outcome or course of a disease; the chance of recovery or recurrence.

At the conclusion of this visit, the doctor will piece together the information you provided at your initial visit, the changes noted on physical exam, and the study results, if the studies were done at the time of, or prior to, this visit. A determination of what further testing will most effectively and safely facilitate arriving at the correct diagnosis will be made based on this information, as well as the results of these tests.

The diagnosis of mesothelioma is definitively confirmed only by a tissue biopsy of the abnormal thickened pleura or the peritoneum.

The diagnosis of mesothelioma is definitively confirmed only by a tissue biopsy of the abnormal thickened pleura or the **peritoneum**; however, cells extracted from fluid and then stained and examined by an expert mesothelioma pathologist or cytologist (specialist who look at tissue/cells under the microscope) can often confirm the diagnosis. With cancers, we make treatment decisions based on an absolutely confirmed diagnosis and no treatment plan, or **prognosis**, will be considered in the absence of a clear-cut pathological diagnosis.

10. Are blood tests useful to diagnose mesothelioma?

There are no blood tests currently approved to directly diagnose mesothelioma. Diagnosis, as stated above, is only confirmed through tissue biopsy with special staining of the tissues, or by means of cytology. These cells can be obtained from an effusion, aspirated from the chest (pleural effusion) or from the abdominal cavity (**ascites**). Some blood tests may be abnormal; for example, elevated **white blood cell (WBC)** count (cells that fight infection), elevated platelet count (cells that aid in the clotting of blood), and the presence of **biomarker** CA 125. These studies are nonspecific and can be found or elevated in non-mesothelioma–related conditions. Mesomark™ has been approved as an experimental test to monitor mesothelioma patients' **response** to therapy, but is not considered appropriate as a diagnostic tool to diagnose the disease itself. It measures a protein called mesothelin, which, in large part, is shed by certain types of mesotheliomas (epithelial, see page 113). This has also become a target for therapy, which we will discuss in Question 66, page 112. Cancers can shed proteins, which may appear in the blood and can be used in some cancers as biomarkers (such as CA-125, noted previously). You might be familiar with the controversial prostate-specific antigen PSA test used to diagnose or assess for the possible presence of prostate cancer. Currently, a number of potential biomarkers of mesothelioma are being studied, but none are approved to diagnose mesothelioma. Scientific advances are occurring so rapidly that it is advisable to constantly look for updates about mesothelioma. The Mesothelioma Applied Research Foundation (Meso Foundation) has unbiased, constantly updated information to assist in keeping you well informed about new developments in regard to both the diagnosis and treatment of mesothelioma.

Ascites

Abnormal build-up of fluid in the abdomen that may cause swelling. In late-stage cancer, tumor cells may be found in the fluid in the abdomen. Ascites is a common manifestation of peritoneal mesothelioma and can occur as a manifestation of recurrent mesothelioma after chest surgery for the disease.

White blood cell (WBC)

Refers to a blood cell that does not contain hemoglobin. White blood cells include lymphocytes, neutrophils, eosinophils, macrophages, and mast cells. These cells are made by bone marrow and help the body fight infection and other diseases.

DIAGNOSIS

Biomarker

A substance some-times found in the blood, other body fluids, or tissues. A high level of bio-marker may mean that a certain type of cancer is in the body. Examples of biomarkers include CA 125 (ovarian can-cer), CA 15-3 (breast cancer), CEA (ovar-ian, lung, breast, pancreas, and gas-trointestinal tract cancers), and PSA (prostate cancer). Also called tumor marker.

Response

The results mea-sured either by X-ray or physical exam of treatment that compares the sta-tus (usually the size) of the tumor before treatment to its sta-tus after treatment.

11. What tests are performed to help diagnose mesothelioma?

One of the first tests ordered is an X-ray. X-rays are easy to perform, are less costly, and can help the pro-vider to determine what other tests will build upon the initial information gained through this test. An X-ray can show fluid both in the abdomen and chest, as well as lung scarring and nodules. Though X-rays are not as sensitive as other tests, they can provide valuable infor-mation early in the process of diagnosing a patient. Another valuable imaging test is a CT (computerized axial tomography) scan, which is more precise in imag-ing an abnormality that may be vague on an X-ray. A dye is injected into one of your veins prior to the pro-cedure and images of your organs and the spaces inside your chest cavity and abdomen can be evaluated in 3D. CT scanning permits the physician to determine the location, size, and shape of any mass or nodule (tumor), and this ability is especially important in arranging a biopsy, as well as monitoring changes in the size and/ or number of tumors in response to a therapy. CT scans can also distinguish between fluid and solid tissue, but they are often not able to distinguish malignant from nonmalignant lymph glands (nodes) or other masses since **lymph nodes** can become secondarily enlarged but not contain malignant cells. Lymph tissue filters fluid that travels through the **lymphatic channels** present in all areas of the body. Lymph nodes play an important role in removing infection or other abnormal particles, such as malignant cells, or organisms from the blood as well as in overall immune response to infections and malignancies. The CT scan also delineates where the tumor is located in relation to other organs, such as the heart, diaphragm (a muscle that is very important in the process of breathing and separates the chest cavity from the abdomen), liver, pancreas, intestines, etc., as well as arteries and veins. Part of the initial **staging**, or extent of the malignant process, is done by means of this CT scan. Staging of the malignancy is important in defining the extent of disease at a given point in time. Staging is important not only in helping to define prognosis (rough estimates of length of survival), but also to suggest treatment options such as surgery or other specialized treatments. We will discuss this staging process in more depth in Part Five.

Magnetic resonance imaging (MRI) is not used as often in mesothelioma as the CT scan, but it can provide valuable information if a tumor is suspected to have invaded adjacent organs, nerves, or bone. This test uses large magnets and computers to display complex images, and importantly, does not involve exposure to any radiation.

Positron emission tomography (PET) scans are especially useful in the staging of mesothelioma, and in identifying patients who may benefit from surgery. The scan relies on identifying tissues that are actively using glucose and measures the amount of this activity. Tumors, cancer cells, and inflamed tissue use more glucose than normal tissue resulting in these areas "lighting up" on the PET scan, but the results of this test need to be interpreted by an expert familiar with mesothelioma as a whole and also especially with regard to and any interventions you may have had. For example, if the PET scan is performed after a surgeon has performed a biopsy, or if a physician has put medicine in your chest to help decrease fluid, there will be areas lighting up due to the inflammation of these procedures, and falsely overestimate the amount of mesothelioma. Small tumor deposits may go undetected by CT scan and the PET

DIAGNOSIS

Lymph node

A rounded mass of lymphatic tissue that is surrounded by a capsule of connective tissue; also called a lymph gland. Lymph nodes filter lymph (lymphatic fluid) and they store lymphocytes (white blood cells). They are located along lymphatic vessels. The involvement of lymph glands by mesothelioma changes the stage to a higher one and is an indication of a more advanced tumor.

Lymphatic channels

Interconnecting tubes that link lymph nodes and allow flow of lymph.

Staging

Performing exams and tests to learn the extent of the cancer within the body, especially whether the disease has spread from the original site to other parts of the body. It is important to know the stage of the disease in order to plan the best treatment.

Magnetic resonance imaging (MRI)

A procedure in which radio waves and a powerful magnet linked to a computer are used to create detailed pictures of areas inside the body; also called nuclear magnetic resonance imaging. These pictures can show the difference between normal and diseased tissue. MRI makes better images of organs and soft tissue than other scanning techniques, such as CT or X-ray. MRI is especially useful for imaging the brain, spine, soft tissue of joints, and insides of bones.

A tissue biopsy usually yields more information about the tumor itself and is more diagnostically reliable than the mere appearance of the cells that is possible when evaluating fluid by means of cytology alone.

scan may be useful in picking up these small primary tumors or deposits of tumors that have developed away from the primary or initial tumor (**metastasis**). Areas that are utilizing glucose in this manner are referred to as hot spots and are quantified by the amount of glucose utilized. PET scans are usually read in relation to an MRI or CT scan, and the latest scans actually fuse PET images with CT or MRI images. Not all insurances cover this type of testing and you will need to inquire with the center performing the test if they have received authorization to do so.

Based upon the results of this testing, a biopsy may be planned.

12. How are biopsies performed, and which biopsy is best for me?

The least invasive procedure that the physician feels will be sufficient to obtain an adequate sample for a pathologist to render an opinion as to the diagnosis is usually chosen. A patient with ascites (fluid in the abdomen) or an effusion (fluid surrounding the lung) may have a procedure performed to remove some or most of that fluid. **Thoracentesis** is the term used to remove fluid from the lung while **paracentesis** is the term used for removing fluid from the abdomen. Samples of these fluids are sent to both the **cytology** laboratory as well as the pathology laboratory to study them for malignant as well as non-malignant conditions. In some cases, fluid alone is able to determine the diagnosis of mesothelioma, but a tissue biopsy usually yields more information about the tumor itself and is more diagnostically reliable than the mere appearance of the cells that is possible when evaluating fluid by means of cytology alone. In specific settings a needle biopsy will be performed by either a radiologist, surgeon, or pulmonologist. The biopsy site is numbed and a large bore needle is used to obtain a specimen. Following any of these procedures, where a needle is introduced into the chest cavity, an X-ray will be obtained to look for any complications such as a **pneumothorax** (air in the chest cavity) or bleeding (hemothorax), and to see if the majority of fluid has been removed and that the lung is expanding properly. Specimens are then sent to the cytologist and pathologist, who will, in addition to evaluating the tissue using only a microscope, stain the tissue using specific stains and antibodies that may help in specifically recognizing certain cancer types including mesothelioma. Once mesothelioma has been diagnosed, based upon the results of the appearance of the tissue as well as these more specific stains and antibody studies, the microscopic appearance of the cells then provides information as to the specific sub-type of mesothelioma you might have and these are referred to as epitheloid, sarcomatoid, or a mixture of the two, which is called mixed or biphasic.

There are situations in which a more invasive procedure is indicated. If an area is too risky or not amendable for a needle biopsy then a more extensive procedure is planned. Sometimes the fluid in the chest or abdomen is **loculated** (walled off into sections by scar tissue), which makes draining the fluid and obtaining random biopsies near impossible. Another scenario leading to a more invasive procedure would be a prior biopsy that did not yield conclusive results or an accumulation of fluid despite a non-diagnostic biopsy. The next level of investigation would be a **thoracoscopy** in which the surgeon inserts a lighted scope with a camera through a small incision in the chest wall. If suspicious areas are identified, biopsies will be taken. This permits the surgeon to

Positron emission tomography (PET) scan

A procedure in which a small amount of radioactive glucose (sugar) is injected into a vein and a scanner is used to make detailed, computerized pictures of areas inside the body where the glucose is used. Because cancer cells often use more glucose than normal cells, the pictures can be used to find cancer cells in the body.

Metastasis

The spread of cancer from one part of the body to another. A tumor formed by cells that have spread is called a metastatic tumor or a metastasis. The metastatic tumor contains cells that are like those in the original (primary) tumor. The plural form of metastasis is metastases (meh-TAS-ta-seez).

Thoracentesis

Removal of fluid from the pleural cavity through a needle inserted between the ribs.

DIAGNOSIS

Paracentesis

Insertion of a thin needle or tube into the abdomen to remove fluid from the peritoneal cavity. Commonly used to make the diagnosis of peritoneal meso-thelioma in patients with ascites or to diagnose recurrence of the disease in the belly.

Cytology

The study and cat-egorization of cells using a microscope.

Pneumothorax

Air within the chest cavity.

Loculated

When fluid in the chest cavity or abdo-men is unable to flow freely. We often used the term "walled off" to mean that the flow is inter-rupted by disease, scar tissue, or thick viscous fluid.

Thoracoscopy

The use of a thin, lighted tube (called an endoscope) to examine the inside of the chest.

Peritoneoscopy

The use of a lapa-roscope, a thick, lighted tube, to examine the abdomen.

obtain multiple biopsies and also to get a more in-depth look within the chest itself. This tissue will then be examined for cancer cells. In making treatment-related decisions the surgeon will have the opportunity during this procedure to identify areas where the disease is located, specifically whether the lung is involved. Crucial decisions can be made based upon the examination as it may very well reveal areas not well imaged on CT scans, MRI, or PET that might impact the type of surgery to be planned or if a surgical option is indeed possible in a particular patient. Of particular concern is whether dis-ease has spread to the lung or diaphragm, whether it is embedded into the chest wall, or whether it has invaded the mediastinum (center of the chest) or attached itself to the pericardium (sac surrounding the heart).

In peritoneal mesothelioma, a **peritoneoscopy** is some-times performed if a patient is thought to have disease not amendable to surgery. The goal of surgery in perito-neal mesothelioma is to completely cytoreduce (remove gross tumor down to very small residual levels), and if patients have bowel involvement or invasion into vital organs, surgery is not thought to be of benefit. Abdomi-nal mesothelioma can be difficult to image on CT scans, MRI, or PET. Therefore having an inside view by peri-toneoscopy can help the surgeon to determine if the patient is operable as well as to alert the surgeon as to the type of problems he or she is likely to encounter.

An open biopsy may be necessary if scans reveal that the area in question has more solid tumor or minimal fluid. This procedure is best performed by an experienced mesothelioma surgeon who will ultimately guide you in making treatment-related decisions, as well as suggest **referrals** to medical and radiation oncologists who also share expertise in the field of mesothelioma treatment.

An experienced surgeon will be thinking ahead and planning to utilize this surgical incision line for a future surgery. Patients will receive general anesthesia and the surgeon will make a small incision 3–4 inches on the side of the chest to allow adequate sampling from the thickened pleura. It may be necessary to remove part of a rib to allow enough space to perform the procedure in order to procure an amply sized piece of pleura (ideally as big or bigger than a dime). When possible, the sample will be directly examined by a pathologist to ensure that it is adequate for making a diagnosis and that enough material was obtained for required testing. The chest cavity is usually not entered during this procedure and often a chest tube (to drain air out of the chest) is not necessary. Patients are prescribed pain medication for the week following this procedure to make them more comfortable as the site heals.

Referral

A seeking out of expert consultation by a primary physician. The expert may or may not be associated with a cancer center.

13. How will I learn about my biopsy results, and how can I be sure the diagnosis is mesothelioma?

Biopsies are sent to a pathologist who will perform the necessary tests to confirm the diagnosis of mesothelioma. The test results are usually ready 4–5 days following your biopsy. You will need to make an appointment to discuss the results of the biopsy. If you are not in a center where they see a lot of mesothelioma, the biopsy might be sent out for an expert review. If the results use the term suspicious for mesothelioma then the diagnosis is not considered to be confirmed and you may need to request that the biopsy be sent to a more experienced center. Your primary doctor may be the one to discuss the results of this biopsy but he or she will assist you in securing the necessary appointments with specialists in this disease.

DIAGNOSIS

Remember: This is only the beginning of your journey. Don't get frustrated; you will continue to gain confidence in navigating the medical systems.

14. I have been given a diagnosis of mesothelioma. Since this is a rare disease, how do I know that my physicians have enough experience with the disease to treat me?

Mesothelioma is a rare disease and many oncologists and surgeons have never seen a mesothelioma patient prior to your visit. You have the right to ask questions to ensure that you are at the right center. It is preferable if your doctor treats at least 50 mesothelioma patients per year. You should ask if your doctors have published about mesothelioma in peer-reviewed journals or participated in mesothelioma **clinical trials** since that is how we judge our peers to be experts in many fields of medicine. If you are not comfortable with the experience of your team, then ask to be referred to an expert. Mesothelioma is a complicated disease and you will greatly benefit from someone who is compassionate as well as knowledgeable. Your primary care doctor should still remain as part of your healthcare team, receiving updates and serving as an ally and advocate for now and for future needs as they develop. Primary care physicians can facilitate the exchange of information and order some of the necessary tests to make your visit with the expert comprehensive.

Clinical trial

A type of research study that uses volunteers to test new methods of screening, prevention, diagnosis, or treatment of a disease. The trial may be carried out in a clinic or other medical facility. Also called a clinical study.

15. Should I get a second opinion?

In rare diseases such as mesothelioma it is considered customary to request a second opinion. You may like your doctor very much, but if he or she is not an expert in this disease you may be doing more harm than good by not seeking a second opinion. Most doctors recognize this as necessary and gratefully send you to an expert. The role of the expert is to make you aware of your treatment options and to help guide you as you decide what is best for you and your family. The Meso Foundation serves as a resource for referrals for second opinions; I suggest that you utilize this service.

In rare diseases such as mesothelioma it is considered customary to request a second opinion.

16. How do I go about getting a second opinion?

It is very important that you check with your insurance policy to ascertain if they cover second opinions. Some **health maintenance organizations (HMOs)** are restrictive and may wish for you to remain within the system. If they do not have a recognized expert you may request that they refer you out of network. Some patients can afford to pay for a second opinion and do so if they are denied this opportunity through insurance. Expert guidance is crucial in being successful in your treatment of mesothelioma and this often involves travel as well as all the inconveniences associated with it. If you have adult children or other family members and friends who wish to help, this is the time to accept their help.

When you call for your appointment, make sure that you have your Medicare card or other insurance information in hand. You will sometimes be directed to an

Health maintenance organization (HMO)

A form of health insurance combining a range of coverages in a group basis. A group of doctors and other medical professionals offer care through the HMO for a flat monthly rate with no deductibles. However, only visits to professionals within the HMO network are covered by the policy. All visits, prescriptions, and other care must be cleared by the HMO in order to be covered. A primary physician within the HMO handles referrals.

office that will take this information over the phone and they will check with your insurance company to make sure that you are covered.

The specialists will require your pathology report and slides. The slides can be requested at the hospital where you had your surgery or biopsy. You will also need your scans and scan reports. The scans will be placed on CDs, making them easy to hand carry or mail depending on the preference of the center where you have your upcoming appointment. If you have had any prior mesothelioma surgery, that report will also be necessary. If you are instructed to mail these reports and slides, do so using a service that provides a tracking number so you can be sure they are not lost in transit. Often your primary care physician will work with the staff of the referring doctor to help facilitate the transfer of materials.

Sarah adds....

I found it to be very helpful to try and plan for the unexpected when we traveled out of state for appointments. I tried to call ahead to the doctor's office to verify the appointment time and date and to also find out if I needed to bring anything specific to the appointment that I might not have been aware of. It can be very frustrating to be away from home and arrive to discover you were supposed to bring the X-rays, reports, etc. I also tried to make sure that we packed enough medications with us in case we needed to stay longer than originally expected. It can be very stressful to be out of town and find you didn't bring enough medications or supplies with you and then you must start making phone calls to your doctor at home to call medications in for you and to find local pharmacies to fill them.

17. Who treats mesothelioma?

Let's presume as we describe the members of your medical team that you have researched and that they are mesothelioma specialists (publish in peer-reviewed journals articles about mesothelioma, see more than 50 patients per year with mesothelioma, and participate in mesothelioma clinical trials).

- **Thoracic surgical oncologists** specialize in the chest and are responsible for the surgical management of pleural (lung) or pericardial (sac surrounding the heart) mesothelioma. The **abdominal surgeon** with a specialty in **oncology** (treatment of cancer) will be the surgeon for peritoneal (abdominal) mesothelioma.

- **Radiation oncologists** are responsible for delivering radiation therapy should this be part of your treatment plan.

- The **medical oncologist** will determine the type of chemotherapy and will be responsible for directing the administration of this treatment.

You will usually begin with either the surgeon or medical oncologist. Most of these experts are situated in comprehensive **cancer centers** where they have a number of expert colleagues to assist in your care. This may include pain specialists, nutritionists, and oncology social workers. They should be able to offer clinical trials as well as inform the patient about the **standard of care** approaches to treatment. You deserve the best and should not settle for any team that does not impress you with their expertise as well as compassion for your current situation. If you are not satisfied you can and should seek additional consultations.

DIAGNOSIS

Thoracic surgical oncologist

A board certified, general thoracic surgeon whose practice is almost exclusively the treatment of cancers in the chest.

Abdominal surgeon

A surgeon who specializes in surgery below the diaphragm.

Oncology

The study of cancer.

Radiation oncologist

A physician who delivers radiation.

Medical oncologist

A specially certified physician who treats cancer and delivers chemotherapy.

Cancer center

A hospital that specializes only in the care of patients with cancer. A National Cancer Institute (NCI)-designated cancer center is specifically recognized and partially funded by the National Cancer Institute.

Standard of care

In medicine, treatment that experts agree is appropriate, accepted, and widely used. Healthcare providers are obligated to provide patients with the standard of care. Also called standard therapy or best practice.

18. How do I find the best doctors to treat my mesothelioma?

The Internet can facilitate your search for a mesothelioma specialist. If you are not computer savvy you can enlist friends and family to assist you in identifying some expert centers. The Resource section lists Web sites and organizations that can assist you in locating a specialist. Your family doctor or internist may have some knowledge of these specialists but it is up to you to do your own research in order to make sure that you are seeing the very best doctors that you can. Do not be afraid to ask questions and to call the offices as well to request additional information. Keep reading as we want to make sure that you are well prepared to ask the right questions and understand the basics of this disease so you can make the best choices and obtain the best possible outcome.

19. What can I do to make my doctor visits as productive as possible?

It is extremely important that the doctor receive all of the reports, scans, and pathology material in advance of your visit. Call ahead to make sure that this is so. On the day of the visit try to be well rested and bring a family member or close friend to provide support and an additional set of ears. Oftentimes many family members wish to accompany you to the visit but limiting the number of people in the room will allow the focus to be on you and your needs. Identify someone who you feel most comfortable with and designate tasks that others can assist you with so they too will feel needed. Take the time to read this book and then formulate questions that you would like to have answered. Initially most doctors will begin by recounting the facts leading up to your diagnosis and summarize your symptoms. We sometimes use medical jargon that is unfamiliar to you. It is perfectly acceptable for you to ask for further clarification of any terminology that you do not understand. Sometimes doctors assume that you have information when in fact you may not have been told some very important facts. Slowly discuss your understanding of the disease and your particular situation. Look at your list of questions and ask any that may not have been discussed up to this point. If you have additional fears and concerns, it is important to begin an honest dialogue with your doctor. He or she will be your most trusted confidant and nothing that you say or wish to discuss will shock them. You may request privacy and have whoever is accompanying you step out of the room. This is *your* visit and the focus needs to be on your needs so feel free to exercise the right to privacy. You should not feel rushed nor should any questions be brushed off. You have the right to expect information and to be informed in a manner that is understandable and complete. Take the time to meet the members of your treatment team and get contact information for all. Most specialists have either nurses or physician assistants who are readily available for follow-up questions.

Sarah adds…

I found that at many of the doctor appointments we would be asked numerous times by people in the office what medications Phil was taking, the dosage, etc. I made a chart listing this information and would give it to the staff and doctor. It saved time and also kept us from repeating the same information over and over again.

Taking a notebook with questions or concerns that you have about the particular treatment plan or test results is helpful so you won't forget to ask them while in the office. It can be difficult to contact the doctor once you leave the office to ask something you may have forgotten. The notebook was also helpful to write down any new information or medical terminology that you're not familiar with so you can do some research on it at home and be prepared for the next meeting to discuss it.

Keeping a list of all the doctor's names and why they were treating Phil was also helpful to have on hand for appointments so that the doctor we were seeing that particular day was aware of these doctors and for which condition they were treating him. It was a way to keep all the doctors aware of what others were doing.

PART THREE

Coping

What types of psychosocial support
are available to me?

What should my family know about
mesothelioma in order to assist me?

What insurance and financial concerns do I need to
address following a mesothelioma diagnosis?

More...

20. What types of psychosocial support are available to me?

A healthcare team is made up of many individuals who can provide support to you. These include doctors, nurses, social workers, counselors, and many other professionals who you may see during your illness. They are all very willing to help you deal with the diagnosis in any way possible. Don't hesitate to call on them when you need to. It is important that you be in your best possible shape when making the difficult decisions that you will need to during the time of this illness and in managing the complications of life with mesothelioma. This implies maintaining your general physical fitness as well as psychological and mental fitness. Admitting that you are having difficulty coping with these challenges facilitates a dialogue with your healthcare team giving them the opportunity to provide you with resources that can assist you.

Support groups allow you to communicate with others who have had similar experiences, and they are an excellent source of information. Unfortunately, because mesothelioma is such a rare disease, there has been a lack of specific support groups for such patients. The Meso Foundation (www.curemeso.org) has regularly scheduled telephone support groups. These support groups are available for patients, caregivers, and those that have lost loved ones to the disease. You are provided a call-in number and passcode to ensure the confidentiality of these calls. Individual counseling is also available from their nurse practitioner, an experienced medical professional who has worked in the field of mesothelioma for more than 15 years. Your doctor and/or the foundation can give you the names and phone numbers of patients with mesothelioma that are undergoing or have undergone treatment and are willing to share their experiences with other individuals diagnosed with mesothelioma. Patients are usually willing and eager to share their experiences with others and may provide excellent support to you. They are able to provide a patient's point of view and share their personal experiences. This enables you to have a better understanding of what the process may be like and what you can expect before treatment even starts.

21. What should my family know about mesothelioma in order to assist me?

Telling family members about your diagnosis is a difficult thing to do. They could experience a lot of the same emotions that you do, including fear, worry, concern, anger, and sadness. These emotions need to be expressed, even when they are strong. The best recommendation is to communicate openly and honestly with one another. This enables you and your family to cope better with the cancer diagnosis. Your entire adult family should discuss all aspects of the disease before you start treatment. This includes the type of mesothelioma, the prognosis, treatment options, goals of treatment, and expected side effects. If a family member has specific questions that cannot be answered within the group or requires more in-depth information, he or she should feel free to call the doctor to discuss these issues, and should understand that the doctor will be happy to inform him or her so that you and your loved ones are on the same wavelength! Your personal consent is required for any member of the healthcare team to discuss your disease specifics with anyone other than yourself. Please make sure that you provide that permission to your healthcare team in writing in advance of any calls from family members or other healthcare supporters and proxies.

COPING

22. What insurance and financial concerns do I need to address following a mesothelioma diagnosis?

When you are faced with a medical diagnosis of cancer, there are many issues that come to the forefront. One important consideration is your insurance coverage. Having healthcare insurance does decrease the financial burden that is placed upon you; however, even with good insurance, out-of-pocket or additional healthcare costs can be high. It is important to find out what your particular insurance plan covers and what you will be held responsible for. All health plans are not created equal in this regard, and the amount you may have to pay can vary widely. Don't assume that something will be paid for without first thoroughly investigating the situation. It is necessary to understand your healthcare policy before starting any treatment plan so that there are no surprises. It is often helpful to obtain an advocate through your insurance agency who can be your point of contact during the course of your illness. Often insurance companies do appoint such a case manager especially in the setting of more complicated and long-term illnesses such as cancer and especially mesothelioma. If you are dissatisfied with your coverage, a social worker at your treating facility or associated with your doctor's office may be able to assist you in understanding what additional options you might have.

23. What should I know about medical records, and how do I manage them?

It is a good idea to keep a personal copy of all your medical records in a file so that you can access them when needed. It becomes difficult to remember everything that has happened to you over the course of your illness, and having these records is a good way to keep things organized. You can obtain a copy of your records by contacting the medical records department of the hospital and/or clinic where you have received, or are currently receiving, treatment. Also, you can request medical records from your doctor's office. To obtain your records, you may have to sign a written request form and pay a fee for the service. You will also want to get copies of all the tests you have had, including laboratory studies and X-ray/CT scan reports. (Today, radiological images can be placed on a CD, which facilitates your being able to carry these records with you from one doctor to another for assessment). This will provide you with a full health history of all your experiences from the time of the diagnosis of your mesothelioma. If you have to see another doctor or specialist at some time in the future, you can bring a copy of your records with you so the new consulting doctor will be more easily able to gain a full understanding of your medical history. You should add to your files a list of the medications you have taken or are currently taking, as well as all the side effects of any or all of these drugs. A copy of your healthcare proxy, medical directives, and DNR (do not resuscitate) instructions should also be kept in this folder. If you do not have a legal form detailing your wishes, arrange one as soon as possible. It is always better to think these things through when you are not in a crisis. Every healthy adult should have healthcare directives to ensure that their wishes are carried out. Your lawyer can assist you in obtaining the forms and ensuring that they are state compliant. Maintaining a sense of direction during this stressful time is imperative, and organization can help maintain that sense of direction and control. Keeping your resources, reports, contacts, and treatment history will help you locate information whenever necessary.

PART FOUR

The Politics of Mesothelioma

Why all the uproar about this disease, and what are the legal implications of having mesothelioma?

How do I learn more about my legal rights regarding mesothelioma?

Do I need to have a will?

More...

24. Why all the uproar about this disease, and what are the legal implications of having mesothelioma?

While mesothelioma is a rare disease, it is found most commonly in people who have been exposed to asbestos. Asbestos was a popular material used for many purposes from the early 1900s through the 1980s. It is rarely used today in the United States but is still readily used in developing countries throughout the world.

Asbestos was used in a variety of products including, among other things, pipe covering, cement, cloth, gaskets, joint compound, floor tiles, shingles, roofing, brake linings, clutches, wire, electrical panels and boards, and safety clothing. Asbestos has also been found to be a contaminant in talc.

Even though asbestos is rarely used in the United States today, it is still ever present. Asbestos-containing materials that were used in ships, buildings, homes automobiles, and numerous other places are often still in place and must be dealt with carefully.

Latency period

The time between the actual exposure to a carcinogen like asbestos and the development of cancer, such as in mesothelioma.

Also, because the **latency period** for developing mesothelioma and other asbestos-related diseases can range from 10 to more than 50 years from the date of first exposure, many people who worked with or were exposed to asbestos many years ago may just be seeing the consequences of such exposure now.

The legal remedy comes from the fact that even though people who were exposed to asbestos years ago did not know of the hazards (or in some cases that they were even using or being exposed to asbestos), companies that manufactured, sold, or used asbestos-containing materials knew or should have known of those hazards and failed to warn or adequately inform the consuming public. Put simply, companies have an obligation to know what is in the products they are manufacturing, selling, and using to keep abreast of any hazards that may result from using such products and to adequately warn consumers of any such dangers.

Indeed, there is ample evidence in the medical and scientific literature that the hazards of asbestos were being discussed and analyzed as early as the beginning of the 20th century. There is also evidence that many companies discussed such dangers in internal corporate documents but did nothing to share that knowledge with the consuming public.

Accordingly, anyone who has been diagnosed with mesothelioma or any other asbestos-related disease should explore their legal rights.

25. I understand that mesothelioma and other asbestos-related diseases are controversial political issues. Why?

Since the beginning of the millennium, the news media, authors, and government agencies and officials have paid increasing attention to asbestos and the diseases it causes.

Likewise, there has been a growing debate regarding the litigation against asbestos manufacturers and the financial impact it has had on those companies and their insurers. There is also growing pressure to address the concerns of the manufacturers and their insurers while not eroding the rights and well being of mesothelioma patients and their families.

Since the early 1900s the truth about asbestos and the diseases it causes has been known—and hidden—from the American public. The United States and Canada are the only remaining western countries that have not yet made significant efforts to halt the use and trade of asbestos. Too many believe that asbestos has been banned or that lengthy, intense exposure is needed to cause illness. Both of those beliefs are myths.

As a mesothelioma victim or as a family member of a victim, you should stay informed regarding these political issues. If you are a union member, union publications may also be a good source of legislative information.

26. I'm finding more and more people whose lives have been affected by mesothelioma. We all agree that we want to do something about this disease. What can be done at the community level?

The staff and volunteers of the Meso Foundation (www.curemeso.org) will gladly assist anyone interested in forming support organizations, raising funds for research, and increasing awareness.

Moreover, it is important to support and thank government officials, whether they are OSHA or EPA staff, members of Congress, or your state legislature who advocate for mesothelioma patients and their families, work to ensure fair and proactive measures to eradicate this disease, and address the medical and personal well being of patients. Enormous pressure is exerted on these public servants regularly aimed at eroding patient and family rights.

Contact your local or area American Cancer Society chapter and medical facilities. Identify yourself as someone who is dealing firsthand with mesothelioma. Ask to be listed as a contact for others who may be dealing with this disease.

Write letters to the editor of local newspapers or other publications when issues surface regarding asbestos. Do what you can to inform the public that asbestos has not been banned and that even brief exposure to asbestos can seriously affect one's health.

Encourage family members and friends to join you in your efforts to increase community awareness and to influence the legislative process.

27. As someone who's been diagnosed with mesothelioma, do my family and I have any legal rights?

Yes. Because mesothelioma is caused by exposure to asbestos, you may be able to recover damages for pain and suffering and loss of life's enjoyment as well as medical costs and lost income, from responsible companies who may have sold, supplied, installed, or manufactured asbestos-containing materials to which you may have been exposed. Your spouse may also be able to recover for what is known as loss of consortium, which includes the loss of a spouse's care, comfort, guidance, and support. Each state has different regulations regarding the timing of bringing an asbestos suit. Accordingly, you should initiate a claim as soon as you are able to do so.

28. How do I learn more about my legal rights regarding mesothelioma?

Mesothelioma is a very specialized disease, and the same way you would want to obtain a physician who specializes in mesothelioma, you should do the same thing when seeking legal consultation. The Internet and social media have become good sources for finding legal specialists. Other sources of information include your doctors, nonprofit research and patient groups such as the Meso Foundation, local or state bar association, and other mesothelioma patients and their families.

Usually attorneys in these types of matters charge what is known as a contingency fee, which is calculated based on a percentage of whatever is recovered in the lawsuit. Accordingly, you should not be required to pay any money up front. Expenses are also usually paid from what is recovered in the lawsuit.

When selecting an attorney, it is important for you to inquire about the extent of his or her experience, knowledge, and success in representing clients with mesothelioma. You need someone who has the resources to fully explore all the possible avenues of your exposure to asbestos and has the ability to follow through in pursuing all the parties responsible for your exposure. Questions to ask would include:

1. How long have you been representing people diagnosed with mesothelioma?
2. How many of your trial lawyers have actually tried mesothelioma cases?

3. Will you be referring my case to another law firm or will your firm handle my case?

4. Has the law firm contributed to or been involved with nonprofit organizations advocating on behalf of mesothelioma patients?

29. Because of the intensity of dealing with the diagnosis, shouldn't I wait with the legal issues and focus first on medical treatments and recovery?

While that would certainly be ideal, mesothelioma is an unpredictable disease. There are also statutes of limitation differing among the states detailing a time frame from the time of diagnosis to the date that your attorney initiates a claim on your behalf. It is best to contact an attorney as soon as you are able and let them begin their end of the process while you concentrate on your medical situation. The information you possess regarding your exposure, including names, dates, and locations, needs to be documented properly and promptly. Considerable research and follow-up is needed for the attorneys to prepare your case. The earlier you make that initial contact and begin the legal process, the better. Attorneys who specialize in mesothelioma-related personal injury cases are very aware of the physical and emotional stresses of the disease and treatments. They will be sensitive and thoughtful in their work on your case, including scheduling meetings and phone conversations, detailing your exposure, and so on.

30. If my case of mesothelioma is due to work-related exposure, am I eligible for workers' compensation?

Perhaps. Your eligibility will depend on the workers' compensation laws in your state. Your attorney can assist you with your workers' compensation questions. It is important to keep in mind that the only remedy you may have against your employer for asbestos exposure would be in a workers' compensation action, which is different than a regular negligence or products liability action that could be brought against manufacturers or suppliers of asbestos-containing products.

31. What types of records might be needed for the legal process?

For work-related exposure, you'll need W-2s and other tax records as well as social security records, and the names, addresses, and phone numbers of work colleagues. For exposure during military service, you'll need your military records. For other types of exposure, the information needed may include the addresses of the site(s) where exposure occurred, the names of others who may be familiar with the exposure, and any products known to contain asbestos. If you are uncertain about the exact source of your exposure, your attorney should have the resources available to do a thorough work and social history to assist you in determining how you may have been exposed.

Medical records confirming your diagnosis as well as your care and treatment are also important documents to be obtained. Most of these records can be obtained by your attorneys once you provide them with a signed authorization.

32. Do I need to have a will?

Because of the nature of mesothelioma as well as the litigation process, a will is strongly recommended. The timing and size of awards and/or settlements of cases are difficult to predict. Having a will that lays out for your loved ones how you wish to have your assets disbursed well in advance of your death will relieve much stress and anxiety for you and for them. In addition, it is important to designate an executor of your estate who would take over as the plaintiff in your lawsuit should you die. An attorney who specializes in wills and estates can assist you and your family in making wise and timely decisions.

PART FIVE

Treatment

What is staging and why is it important?

What are the survival rates for mesothelioma?

What, in general, are the treatment options
for mesothelioma?

More...

33. I have been successful in being referred to a mesothelioma treatment center. What can I expect now?

Once your insurance has been verified and an appointment date is set, an exchange of information takes place. The expert will need to have full copies of your mesothelioma record. This normally includes all scans, reports of surgical procedures, and pathology reports together with the slides of tissue from which the pathological diagnosis of your mesothelioma was made. We usually suggest that you follow up with the expert's office a few days before the appointment, to make sure that all the information and pathological specimens they requested have been received. You may still have time to hand carry anything that was not sent in advance. The initial consultation will include a comprehensive physical exam as well as a review of your current and past medical history. Most patients will have already had a series of X-rays and scans performed, which will be reviewed by the expert and his team at this appointment. Following this comprehensive review, the consultative part of this visit will begin. It is not uncommon for the expert to ask, "What do you know about your diagnosis?" This question provides an opportunity to clarify any misperceptions you may have about the disease from other sources, for example generalists, media, and the web. You can then expect to be educated about mesothelioma on a more personalized basis. In this book, we discuss statistics and generalizable information, which provides the groundwork for this discussion, as well as assisting you in becoming familiar with some of the technical terms and medical jargon that will now be incorporated into your vocabulary. Where you fit into the statistics and what is known about the disease will be a key aspect of the discussion with the expert.

When you see an expert, he or she will have a wealth of knowledge gained by treating others who many have presented to them in a very similar fashion to yourself. This collective wisdom, usually attained over the years, combined with their expert understanding of the disease process and treatment options will greatly impact how successful you will be in managing this disease. Treatment options will be discussed and the benefits and risks should be clearly outlined. If there are clinical trials that you might qualify for, these will be discussed in addition to the standard therapeutic options.

A prognosis is not always possible, for much will depend on your response to treatment and/or surgery. We can certainly discuss survival curves and response expectations based on review of the literature and prior patients, but many patients far exceed textbook predictions of survival. Your wishes should also be discussed and sometimes you may need your support team to step outside, should you wish to discuss areas that you wish to remain private between you and your treating physician. You should also expect to be introduced to additional members of the healthcare team. We suggest that you take a card from each person and ask them to describe their role and how they will be involved in your care. There should be a point person that you will be able to contact with additional questions or to clarify the next steps as you proceed with your treatment plan.

Sarah Ann adds…

Getting a card from various members of the medical teams can be a great help. Fortunately, we had a card from the nurse that schedules at the VA, and I was able to call this nurse to track down why tests the doctor wanted had not been scheduled for my dad. The VA system can get difficult to maneuver around because sometimes one hand doesn't seem to know what the other hand is doing. Knowing who to contact for what purpose saves times. When you are being introduced to members of the healthcare team, remember to ask them what their roles are in your patient's care and how best to contact them. Some respond better to emails and some to phone.

34. Who are the members of my healthcare team?

- Medical oncologist: a medical doctor who spends additional years training to care for patients with cancer. Most medical oncologists are board certified in oncology, which requires intensive clinical training and a written exam for certification, which denotes expertise in cancer.

- **Surgical oncologist**: a surgeon who specialized in operating on patients with cancer. A surgical oncology fellowship is an additional 3 years of training following a general surgical fellowship. Some experts will be listed as thoracic surgeons, peritoneal surgeons and/or cardiac thoracic surgeons. We will discuss how to choose a mesothelioma surgeon on page 63 as well as the surgical aspects of mesothelioma care in Questions 44-49.

- Radiation oncologist: a doctor who specializes in giving radiation therapy to cancer patients. Radiation oncologists are board certified and undergo additional years of training. There are many forms of radiation therapy and radiation oncologists will work closely with your medical oncologist and surgical oncologist as their therapy may be complementary to chemotherapy and/or surgery, and its precise timing may need to be carefully coordinated with these other experts on your healthcare team.

Surgical oncologist

A surgeon who specializes in cancer surgery. This surgeon will perform your surgical biopsies and other operative procedures that may be required for your cancer.

Fellow

A doctor who extends his or her medical training in a particular area of medicine such as surgery, medical oncology, and radiology.

- **Fellow** (medical oncology, surgical, or radiation oncology): a qualified doctor who is now in training to specialize in surgery, medical oncology, radiation therapy, etc. You may initially be seen by a fellow who will then report his or her findings to the attending (a doctor responsible for his or her training). Many mesothelioma experts have fellows assigned to them that they train and who may have a specific interest in mesothelioma.

- **Nurse practitioner (NP)/Physician assistant (PA)**: a registered nurse who has undergone additional clinical and educational training, which enables them to work in close collaboration with a specific member of the team (e.g., medical oncologist, surgeon, radiation therapist), as well as act as a liaison between the various medical and ancillary members of the team. NPs and/or PAs will see you in clinic and work closely with your oncologist, surgeon, radiation therapist, etc. They have full prescriptive privileges and assist in maintaining the level of care necessary in the management of patients with complex medical problems.

- **Research nurse**: a nurse whose primary responsibility is to protect study participants and to ensure that the research project is carried out according to the plan approved by the Institutional Review Board (IRB). The nurse will work closely with your physician and assists in obtaining crucial data to ensure that high quality data will ultimately form the basis of academic publications and potentially lead to the development of new treatments in mesothelioma and other malignancies.

Nurse practitioner (NP)

Registered nurses who are prepared through advanced education and clinical training to provide a wide range of preventive and acute healthcare services to individuals of all ages. NPs complete graduate-level education preparation that leads to a master's degree. They have prescriptive authority and work in collaboration with their physician colleagues.

Physician assistant (PA)

A licensed professional who works under the supervision of a physician. They have prescriptive authority and work in a collaborative manner with their physician colleagues.

Research nurse

A nurse who is responsible for ensuring that a clinical trial is conducted according to standard regulated by the protocol sponsors and institutional review board.

35. What is staging and why is it important?

Staging is the medical term used to describe the amount of disease found in your body. Staging is important at the time of your initial diagnosis as well as following any treatment intervention, as all decisions relating to the nature of treatment are made based on the stage of the disease. Unlike lung cancer, mesothelioma does not usually have one predominant mass, but can typically affect many areas that line the chest, lungs, and/or abdominal cavity. In addition to involving many areas, the degree of thickening can vary, thus making it difficult to quantify exactly how much cancer is present. For pleural mesothelioma, we currently use the **International Mesothelioma Interest Group (IMIG) Staging** or the **Brigham and Women's Hospital Staging**, which takes into account the extent of the tumor (T), involvement and location of lymph nodes (N), and if there is metastatic disease (M). This system is not used for peritoneal or pericardial mesothelioma. Mesothelioma is never staged based on plain X-rays, but relies on information gleaned from CT scans and/or MRIs. PET is often used to acquire additional information not easily disclosed by either an MRI or CT scan. (Please refer to Question 11 on page 18 for descriptions of these scans). The most accurate staging takes place during a surgical intervention, such as a thoracoscopy, in which the surgeon is able to get a good look inside your chest and biopsy areas that may be only suspicious.

Lymph nodes are small bean-shaped areas of tissue. The presence or absence of disease affecting the lymph nodes in and around areas of your disease is an important aspect of the staging process, especially during initial planning, as this can influence the decision to operate.

International Mesothelioma Interest Group (IMIG) Staging

A way of defining the size of the tumor and the locations in a uniform way that facilitates comparing groups of patients who undergo medical interventions. This is the most widely used staging system and is currently under review to be updated in the near future.

The most accurate staging takes place during a surgical intervention, such as a thoracoscopy, in which the surgeon is able to get a good look inside your chest and biopsy areas that may be only suspicious.

If a lymph node is cancerous but is found in the operative field, it will be removed at the time of surgery. If lymph nodes that are at a distance from the planned surgical field are affected or thought to be affected by cancer, a patient may not be considered to be an ideal surgical candidate and will be referred for other treatment modalities.

Lymph nodes can be enlarged for many reasons unrelated to cancer, so we often need to have an additional biopsy performed in order to gain the necessary information regarding the lymph nodes in question. If they are located in the center of the chest, a **mediastinoscopy** is performed. This is a relatively minor procedure and is often performed prior to making a final decision to operate even if no obviously enlarged lymph nodes are noted in that area. The key issue for surgery is that the tumor is reduced to levels that cannot be seen, and if this is not possible due to the presence of disease in relatively inaccessible areas of the lungs, chest, or other parts of the body, the decision to proceed with surgery as an initial modality of therapy might need to be reconsidered.

On the other hand, there are circumstances in which surgery, even if it is anticipated that the entire tumor is not going to be removable, will nevertheless need to be undertaken. However, this is usually in settings in which the surgical procedure is being used to relieve some significant medical problem that is preventing you from having a better quality of life. Rarely is surgery indicated in mesothelioma unless a good reduction of the burden of disease can be performed.

In the future, we hope to be able to characterize how aggressive the tumors are and to provide more accurate predictions of the response to a therapy based on

Brigham and Women's Hospital Staging

Process developed at the Brigham and Women's Hospital to better define stage as it relates to surgery. It is meant to offer a better picture of what the expected outcome might be following chest surgery for mesothelioma.

Mediastinoscopy

A procedure to view the organs and structures in the area between the lungs where lymph nodes reside. The tube is inserted through an incision above the breastbone. This procedure is usually performed to get a tissue sample from the lymph nodes on the right side of the chest.

Rarely is surgery indicated in mesothelioma unless a good reduction of the burden of disease can be performed.

the molecular characteristics of the biopsy sample. In early-stage breast cancer, we are already able to do so. In mesothelioma, scientists are furiously searching for markers that will similarly make this a reality, thus enabling a more personalized treatment plan.

36. What are the stages of mesothelioma based on the IMIG Staging System?

Stage Ia: a mesothelioma found on one side of the chest in the lining of the chest wall. It can also be found in the lining of the chest cavity between the lungs and/or the lining that covers the diaphragm. The visceral pleura of the lungs must be unaffected at this time in order for your disease to qualify in this early stage of disease.

Stage Ib: a mesothelioma found in one side of the chest in the lining of the chest wall and the lining that covers the lung. It can also be found in the lining of the chest cavity between the lungs and/or the lining that covers the diaphragm.

Stage II: a mesothelioma that has spread to both layers of the pleura on one side of the body, and has enlarged to form a tumor mass on the pleural tissue around the lung tissue or diaphragmatic muscle.

Stage III: a mesothelioma that has spread to the chest wall or the covering of the heart. It may have also already spread to lymph nodes, but only to those on the same side of the chest, such that the tumor remains surgically resectable.

Stage IV: a mesothelioma in which the disease is widespread (both sides of the chest or the lymph nodes in the mediastinum are affected) or it has invaded other organs. In this situation, it is clearly not feasible to surgically resect the tumor.

37. How does mesothelioma spread?

In general most cancers, including mesothelioma, can spread by direct invasion or via the lymphatic channels through lymph node involvement. Mesothelioma rarely spreads to the central nervous system, but tends to grow in the cavity where it first began. Pleural mesothelioma can grow to completely encase the lung and ultimately spread across the chest involving the esophagus, heart, and opposite lung. In patients who undergo **extrapleural pneumonectomy**, 25% will have the disease return in the abdomen. Peritoneal mesothelioma can become widespread in the abdominal cavity eventually invading the bowel, liver, and other vital organs. Patients will rarely die of mesothelioma itself, but rather from the complications caused by the disease, such as pneumonia, other infections, congestive heart failure, or other organ failure due to invading disease or obstruction.

Mesothelioma rarely spreads to the central nervous system but tends to grow in the cavity where it first began.

Extrapleural pneumonectomy

Surgery to remove a diseased lung, part of the pericardium (membrane covering the heart), part of the diaphragm (muscle between the lungs and the abdomen), and part of the parietal pleura (membrane lining the chest). This type of surgery is used most often to treat malignant mesothelioma.

38. What is my prognosis?

A prognosis is based on gathering credible information about your tumor and your general health. This information includes the size and location of your tumor in addition to the areas it may have spread to, the molecular and pathological features of the tumor (how it looks under the microscope), and how you respond to treatment, be it surgery, chemotherapy, or radiation therapy.

All of these issues are taken into account to determine what your prognosis might be. Although we cannot cure mesothelioma, some patients can live for a relatively long time with an excellent quality of life. Some patients, on the other hand, may not do as well and may be resistant to any form of medical intervention. We have found that patients in the early stages of the disease with epithelial histology and in good health, despite their mesothelioma, tend to fare better than others. For reasons unknown at the present time, women tend to do better than men. It is known that a patients' blood count may also impact on their prognosis. An elevated white blood count (cells that fight infection), elevated platelet count (cells that are responsible for clotting), and low hemoglobin (reflecting the number of red cells that transport oxygen) are poor prognostic factors. Physical fitness, with few if any other medical problems, and being young rather than old also works in your favor to improve your prognosis.

Supportive care

Care given to improve the quality of life of patients who have a serious or life-threatening disease; also called palliative care, comfort care, and symptom management. The goal of supportive care is to prevent or treat as early as possible the symptoms of the disease, side effects caused by treatment of the disease, and psychological, social, and spiritual problems related to the disease or its treatment.

39. What are the survival rates for mesothelioma?

Patients who chose not to be treated or who are unable to undergo treatment have a life expectancy of four to nine months following diagnosis. This can vary, however, based on some of the more favorable characteristics mentioned in Question 38. Some patients opt to have **supportive care** only, which involves treating only their symptoms. Supportive care results in about 50% of these patients surviving beyond 6 months. It has been reported that patients who participate in clinical trials survive longer than patients who chose not to participate. Patients who meet the criteria to be enrolled in clinical trials that use multiple treatments (multimodal trials, described in Question 42), tend to survive longer, and 50% of these patients live 8–18 months after treatment.

As a patient, however, you must realize that you are an individual case, and there are many factors that add up to define these statistics, making it almost impossible to truly predict what your actual survival will be. For example, if you were diagnosed very early and have disease only on the parietal pleura, your chance for long-term survival is much better, with 70% of these patients living for 5 years or longer. However, once the disease involves the surface of the lung, even without invading it (although still stage I if the lymph nodes are not involved), the survival rate decreases to a 30% chance of living for five years. This is by way of illustrating that we are talking about larger groups of people in order to define these rather complex statistical outcomes, none of which may be specific enough to mirror what your survival expectation might be. In addition to all of these imponderables, there is the question as to how treatment will impact on the extent of your disease and thus, your overall survival. As treatments improve, these statistics are likely to change considerably. It takes time, however, for the outcome of new treatments to become statistically apparent, so for now we have only these rather dismal numbers to go by.

By no means does this need to be what you might expect to happen in your case as a lot will ultimately depend on the nature of your treatment, making all accurate predictions impossible.

As a patient, however, you must realize that you are an individual case, and there are many factors that add up to define these statistics, making it almost impossible to truly predict what your actual survival will be.

We are talking about larger groups of people in order to define these rather complex statistical outcomes, none of which may be specific enough to mirror what your survival expectation might be.

40. What do these scary survival rates mean to me as a patient?

Patients can choose to accept these statistics or to explore cutting edge treatments that may extend survival. The field of mesothelioma research is growing at a rapid pace and some of the standard treatments that you are being offered today did not exist 5 years ago. Each patient is an individual and each patient responds to treatment differently. The best way to survive this disease is to stay informed and to protect your general health by eating well, staying hydrated, exercising to the extent that you are able, and constantly maintaining a healthy and positive outlook. Consult a specialist and be willing to travel outside of your comfort zone to seek the best advice and consider participating in cutting-edge treatments where they seem appropriate.

Sarah adds...

I am a firm believer in getting all the information that is available and then making my decisions. Survival rates and statistics were not as important to me as I know that not all cases are alike. You make your decisions based upon your personal experience and understanding of the current situation, as well as current and past medical history.

41. What is palliative care?

Another area that is increasingly being recognized as crucial in cancer care is the field of **palliative care**. Palliative care refers to care focused on relieving problems that are caused by the cancer itself, the resolution of which will not improve your survival but will allow you to live with a better quality of life during the time you are going to survive. This may involve the treatment of

Palliative care

Care directed toward the symptoms related to your cancer diagnosis. Palliative care is usually delivered by a team of trained professionals and can help with symptoms related to spiritual, physical, or emotional distress. The focus is not on your response to treatment but on your ability to carry out and enjoy your daily activities.

pain and/or the stress associated with your cancer, or the treatment of low hemoglobin that may make you tired. People often confuse palliative care with hospice, but the goals of therapy are quite different. **Hospice** is for end-of-life care aimed at easing the suffering of the dying patient and his or her family, thus making the process of dying less stressful for all. Palliative care works in conjunction with your medical therapy to support and assist you in living with the best possible quality of life while you undergo the often rigorous treatments necessary to combat your disease. The palliative care team consists of experts from a myriad of fields who join together to support you during this time. Decision-making is hindered when a patient is suffering from anxiety, depression, fatigue, and pain, so controlling these symptoms will enable you to direct your attention to making the necessary important decisions that will impact upon your survival. Most university hospitals have a palliative care team and you can ask to be referred to their services. They can generally consult with you both inside and outside the hospital setting.

Hospice

A program that provides special care for people who are near the end of life and for their families, either at home, in freestanding facilities, or within hospitals.

Or, as indicated before, palliative care may replace specific cancer-related therapy in settings in which such therapy may do more harm than good, or all therapeutic options have been exhausted, or an individual just chooses not to be treated. The goal again is not to make the dying process easier (hospice care), as is the common misconception about palliative care, but your ongoing living, even in the absence of any treatment that may prolong your life, better.

One of the most common symptoms of mesothelioma is shortness of breath. In many cases, this is brought about by fluid that gets trapped in the pleural space. A chest tube can be inserted through which the fluid is

Drainage of pleural effusion and inserting talc is reserved for patients who are not likely to undergo a more definitive surgical resection, as it makes the surgery more difficult and can also impact the type of surgery we are able to perform.

Catheter

A tube that can be used to drain urine from the bladder; an intravenous catheter is used to give fluids in the vein.

PleurX catheter

Refers to a tube that is inserted into the chest or abdomen allowing fluid to be drained in the comfort of your home. Patients and their caregivers are trained in how to drain these catheters, which has a low complication rate and is really quite simple.

drained and talc instilled into the space in an attempt to prevent further re-accumulation of the fluid. We like to reserve this maneuver for patients who are not likely to undergo a more definitive surgical resection, as it makes the surgery more difficult and can also impact the type of surgery we are able to perform. We also discourage this for patients who may wish to consider some of the new clinical trials, which require access to the pleural space to administer treatment. An alternative approach to remove this fluid may be the placement of a specific **catheter** called the **PleurX catheter**. This is an extremely small catheter that can be inserted into the pleural space without the need for the instillation of talc or other abrasive substances that alter the surgical field. Patients and their care providers are then taught how to drain the fluid through one of these catheters, which can be left in place for many weeks or even months as ongoing treatment allows the preparation of the patient for a more definitive surgical procedure. This approach provides the individual an increased level of freedom in that the patient can manage this process while at home. It is also an effective way of managing recurring fluid problems. Although at first draining the fluid may be a bit unnerving, it is a convenient and safe way to keep the patient comfortable without added trips to and from the clinic or hospital.

Chest pain is another symptom that may require intervention by the healthcare team. Treatment may include **narcotic** medications either by mouth or injection, or a surgical block may be considered if this approach does not work effectively or the side effects from the medication become too significant (constipation, drowsiness, confusion). A nerve block relieves pain by injecting a substance into or around a nerve that could permanently or temporarily destroy that nerve that affects a specific and localized region of your body. Alternatively, a pump can be inserted either to inject narcotics continuously into a subcutaneous area of your body or even into the fluid surrounding the spinal cord in order to adequately control your pain. In some cases, even radiation therapy can be effective in alleviating pain by shrinking a tumor that may be pressing on a specific nerve, but this is dependent on the location being amenable to receiving this therapy.

Chest pain

Discomfort in the chest that can range from a feeling of heaviness to a constant boring pain that requires narcotics.

Narcotic

An agent that causes insensibility or stupor; usually refers to opioids given to relieve pain.

42. What, in general, are the treatment options for mesothelioma?

For patients who wish to actively treat their disease, a number of treatment options are available. Patients who have disease that is considered amendable for surgery will often be offered a multimodality (using many treatment options at once or sequentially) approach, which involves **chemotherapy**, surgery, and radiation. Once you have been evaluated by an expert, a more personalized approach will be initiated. Some surgeons prefer that patients have **neo-adjuvant chemotherapy** (chemotherapy given prior to a surgical intervention with the intent of decreasing the size or local infiltration of the tumor, thus making its resection easier or more feasible). Some surgeons will suggest taking the patient directly to surgery with chemotherapy planned following a short recovery period. Patients who have an extrapleural pneumonectomy (EPP) generally have radiation to the chest cavity following recovery. Patients who have a **pleurectomy decortication (PD)** may not always be referred for radiation therapy. (These two procedures will be discussed in full detail shortly).

Chemotherapy

Treatment with anti-cancer drugs. There are many varieties of these drugs that have different mechanisms for killing cancer cells.

Neo-adjuvant chemotherapy

Chemotherapy that is delivered before a planned surgical or radiation-based treatment.

Pleurectomy/ decortication (PD)

An operation for mesothelioma that removes the involved pleura and frees the underlying lung so that it can expand and fill the pleural cavity.

Multimodality treatment

Therapy that combines more than one method of treatment.

Multimodality treatment is certainly a more aggressive approach than surgery as a single entity. This approach, however, is justified because clinical trials suggest that multimodality treatment translates into a longer survival, especially if a response to therapy is documented prior to surgery. Patients must be carefully evaluated prior to surgery to make sure they are otherwise healthy enough to tolerate such therapy. Your doctors want to ensure that the benefits outweigh the potential harms of an aggressive surgical procedure together with the required chemotherapy and/or radiation. Question 45 discusses what such a **workup** involves in defining your ability to tolerate this approach. It is really the experience of your team in having treated many patients with this multimodality approach that helps them know who may or may not be a candidate for such treatment. Nevertheless, there is more than the testing to define who may be appropriate for this approach and for that reason, the evaluation should be performed by someone who has extensive knowledge and experience in caring for patients with mesothelioma and not just any surgeon or medical oncologist.

Workup

A series of tests to discover information about the patient, most commonly to define extent of disease or suitability for a given treatment.

The goal of surgery is to remove all visible evidence of disease.

The goal of surgery is to remove all visible evidence of disease. We know that cancer cells may escape during and often prior to surgery so the intent of the chemotherapy, in circumstances in which surgery is thought to be complete, is to chase down these cells and prevent them from seeding a new area or allowing the original area to recur. Chemotherapy is a systemic approach to cancer, while radiation therapy is a more localized approach. We use radiation therapy in an attempt to eradicate microscopic disease (not visible to the human eye) that may remain immediately adjacent to or at the surgical site.

In the past, a patient undergoing this surgery was at high risk for complications and even death. Today, experienced mesothelioma surgeons can perform these surgeries with fewer complications and less operative mortality. This is a further compelling reason to seek an experienced specific mesothelioma surgeon who has published his or her results in peer-reviewed journals. Anyone can claim to be an expert or to have the expertise required to perform these procedures, even if they have not done many procedures, but having published results in such journals indicates that the results reported have been accepted as accurate by medical professionals in a prescribed review process. This also indicates a level of expertise that is above that which might be attained by a surgeon who performs only a few of these procedures, and who would thus be unable to gather sufficient data required to publish his or her experience.

If a patient is unable to receive or chooses to not have surgery, he or she may receive chemotherapy alone. The effectiveness of the chemotherapy drugs that have been available in the past was poor. With the development of new agents, however, tumor responses to chemotherapy have improved significantly. However, we remain dissatisfied with our present results, despite the doubling of response rates. As a result, newer agents and combinations of older and newer drugs are constantly being tested to improve on the response rates to increase the number of patients who benefit from therapy.

This is a further compelling reason to seek an experienced specific mesothelioma surgeon who has published his or her results in peer-reviewed journals.

TREATMENT

43. What is performance status, and why is it important?

In order to convey to other doctors the status of a particular patient, we need to have a conventional and standard manner by which each individual can be measured so that even if we do not see the patient, we understand what the status of that patient might be. **Performance status** is used to address the functional status of an individual so that a doctor can estimate whether a patient can withstand specific treatments. The performance status is thus a measure of a person's overall state of health. We use this measure to determine if a patient is fit enough to receive chemotherapy, take part in a clinical trial, or be considered for any or specific surgical procedures. There are two scales currently in use and both measure a patient's level of activity. The best performance, 0–1, describes a patient as being physically able to perform all activities of daily living with few (PS 1) or no (PS 0) symptoms of the disease. Four is the poorest score, reflective of a seriously ill patient who is essentially bedridden and unable to care for him- or herself. We use these scales to assist us in choosing the most appropriate treatment for an individual patient.

Performance status

A measure of how well a patient is able to perform ordinary tasks and carry out daily activities.

44. What surgery is performed for mesothelioma?

There are a number of surgical options for patients with pleural mesothelioma. As we discussed earlier, many patients with pleural mesothelioma initially present with shortness of breath and a pleural effusion. We may initially investigate the patient's symptoms using a thoracoscopic procedure. Thoracoscopy involves one to three small incisions, usually one for a camera, and two for using instruments to biopsy or retract. This enables us to obtain biopsies, as well as to look inside the chest to assist in decision-making for future surgery. Patients with fluid will have a chest tube inserted to drain the fluid and in those patients who have already been determined to not be surgical candidates, the surgeon can instill talc as a means to prevent the fluid from returning. Experienced centers will refrain from using talc in a patient who might be considered for surgery, but if you have had this procedure before seeing a mesothelioma specialist, it makes the surgery more difficult but not impossible.

A pleurectomy decortication (PD) is a procedure in which both the linings of one lung are removed — that is both the visceral and parietal pleura. An extrapleural pneumonectomy (EPP) is a procedure in which the entire lung, as well as portions of the diaphragm and pericardial sac, is removed. The pleural surfaces are also removed as part of this more extensive surgery. These are complex surgeries and not only does it take an advanced level of skill to perform them, but additional expertise, specifically in the setting of mesothelioma, is crucial in determining what type of procedure is best suited for you.

In peritoneal mesothelioma, the standard operation is referred to as a **debulking procedure**. In this surgery, all visible evidence of disease is removed. In many circumstances at the conclusion of the surgery today, the abdomen is treated with chemotherapy, heated and infused directly into the all the crevices of abdominal space, which might have been contaminated by single mesothelioma cells. This is a specialized type of surgery and treatment and should only be performed in centers with vast experience in treating peritoneal mesothelioma, as the surgery may often entail the removal of parts of

Debulking procedure

The removal of as much disease as possible with the goal of leaving only microscopic disease behind that is invisible to the naked eye.

the bowel and/or other organs, which requires a level of expertise that is not attainable by all standard surgeons or even surgical oncologists.

45. What determines whether I am able to have surgery?

A full medical checkup is necessary to determine if you are healthy enough to have any of the surgical procedures described previously. The surgeon will want to know if you have any heart, lung, kidney, or liver problems that may preclude you from undergoing a lengthy period of anesthesia and recovery. This is determined by a general and full clinical examination usually performed by the medical oncologist who knows what specific features to look for that may indicate an individual's ability to withstand, or not withstand, any of these procedures. Again, this requires an experienced team who has guided many patients through these procedures, and which can determine if an individual may not be an ideal candidate. Additionally, specific laboratory testing, including electrocardiogram (EKG), **pulmonary function tests**, cardiac ultrasound, and blood testing, will be performed in order to confirm your status and to define issues that might require correction prior to your undergoing surgery. Underlying blood abnormalities should be corrected so as to minimize their impact on the procedure, such as problems that may lead to excessive bleeding, clot formation during or after surgery, or anemia that may delay or impair healing. We spoke earlier about performance status; this is an overall assessment of your clinical status and thus a general determination of how you will tolerate and recover from any of these surgical procedures.

Pulmonary function test

A series of breathing maneuvers performed in a certified laboratory that measures the lung capacity and the force with which an individual can inhale and exhale.

In order for surgery to be contemplated as an initial form of treatment, your disease must be confined to one side of the chest or, in the setting of a peritoneal mesothelioma, only in the abdominal cavity. Surgery is not without risk and we wish to operate on only those patients who we think will benefit from these procedures, especially the specific aggressive approaches used by mesothelioma surgeons, and refrain from operating on those patients who may not benefit and indeed may suffer more if operated upon.

46. What determines which surgical procedure I will have?

You will have a full consultation with the surgeon who will evaluate all of your medical data as well as your current state of health. Most specialized mesothelioma surgeons take a very individualized approach, as one size *does not* fit all. In this initial meeting, the goal of the surgery will be discussed. We use surgery to control symptoms, to deliver a new type of therapy that can only be done in the operating room such as the exposure of the abdomen to being bathed with a **heated perfusion** of chemotherapy, or as part of a multimodality treatment course and not specifically as a means of removing all of the tumor. If you have elected to participate in a clinical trial, then the type of surgery is predetermined and hopefully can be carried out as planned. If you are not able to undergo that specific surgery or do not want to undergo that surgical procedure, then clearly you will not be able to proceed with that clinical trial. Your preference as to which surgical procedure you wish to undergo will certainly be taken into account, but the reality is that in many instances the final decision, regarding the extent and type of procedure, takes place

Heated perfusion
The delivery of heated chemotherapy chemicals to the chest and/or abdomen in the operating room after the majority of the tumor is removed.

Your preference as to which surgical procedure you wish to undergo will certainly be taken into account, but the reality is that in many instances the final decision, regarding the extent and type of procedure, takes place in the operating room.

in the operating room. A CT scan can help to guide the surgeon, but mesothelioma is best staged when the surgeon has your chest open and can get a good view of the area(s) involved. Not infrequently, the CT and PET scans prove inadequate at assessing the extent of disease so that a change in the plan may have to be made when the realities of what is present are found at the time of surgery, thus forcing the surgeon's hands or even resulting in the cancellation of any resection. Each surgeon may have his or her own preferences as well, which is a further compelling reason for seeking an experienced mesothelioma surgeon. These surgeons know the data associated with the results of specific surgical procedures in the setting of mesothelioma as opposed to other tumors, and will take these data into consideration when deciding on the best approach to be taken in your specific case. Importantly, such an experienced mesothelioma surgeon also has his or her own past experience, which may sway his or her thoughts about which procedure to perform based on an educated opinion as to what would be in your best interest, as opposed to what might be considered the most appropriate course of action by someone following the standard of care practices who is unfamiliar with the nuances of care necessary in the setting of mesothelioma.

Despite our best efforts, to date, it is extraordinarily difficult to cure mesothelioma. Therefore, in deciding on the most appropriate *type* of surgery, we must also consider relapse patterns based on the individual characteristics of your disease compared to large cohorts of patients who have been operated on in the past. The goal is to render you free of macroscopic disease (disease that is visible to the human eye), while exposing you to the fewest risks possible. Sometimes we have no choice, in that the disease is too bulky for a simple PD and we must plan on an EPP. Some surgeons, on the other hand, prefer to do an EPP if at all possible, regardless of the circumstances, and do not feel that a PD can accomplish the same result in terms of removing macroscopic disease.

This argument over which is the best surgical procedure remains one of the most controversial and emotionally debated aspects of the treatment of mesothelioma. The decision process becomes even more controversial in cases of **early mesothelioma**, in which there is minimal or no involvement of the lung and the disease is primarily on the parietal pleura. All thoracic surgeons agree that performing an EPP can have long-term health implications for the patient. Unfortunately there are no data specifically comparing one operation to the other in this setting of early-stage disease, making it difficult to decide whether doing an EPP, regardless of the extent of disease, is advantageous to a majority of patients, despite the problems associated with immediate postoperative recovery as well as possible longer-term respiratory issues.

Another complicating issue is the use of talc and other material placed into the chest at the time that the diagnosis is made and in the presence of a pleural effusion in order to prevent further fluid accumulation. A common scenario occurs when a patient has a lot of fluid but minimal solid tumor, most of which is on the inner lining of the chest. If that patient has talc or other material added to the chest cavity, thus cementing the lung to the chest wall, this may severely affect the chance for an EPP.

All of this suggests that the patient must take an active role and ask the tough questions. We all understand that statistics are just the law of averages and may not predict

Early mesothelioma

Mesothelioma discovered before the onset of major symptoms. For example, patients may be undergoing a routine procedure when mesothelioma is found without any suspicion of a malignancy, and usually the disease is limited to a single cavity with no evidence of distant spread or lymph node involvement.

All of this suggests that the patient must take an active role and ask the tough questions.

TREATMENT

how you will fare, but they do provide the foundation for a frank discussion with the surgeon. You must also consider how much of a risk *you* are willing to take. This is your decision, and it would be unfair to ask your family to make this decision for you. You need to establish a trusting relationship with your medical team and reach an understanding concerning the possibility that the surgery planned may not be the surgery performed. In a **protocol**, the type of surgery is most often dictated but in non-protocol situations, you do have the right to set parameters for what can be done. If you feel strongly about a PD versus an EPP, you can be very clear when consenting to surgery. The best-case scenario is that you have chosen a surgeon that you trust and value their years of experience and thus their ability to make these tough decisions based on what they encounter in the operating room. If not, perhaps you need to get a second surgical opinion. Only in this way will you be able to confidently move forward with a plan that is based on the knowledge you have garnered and that seems to you and your family to represent the best option for your care.

Protocol

An action plan for a clinical trial. The plan states what the study will do and how and why it will do it. It explains how many people will be in it, who is eligible to participate, what study agents or other interventions they will be given, what tests they will receive and how often, and what information will be gathered.

47. What can I expect before surgery, and what can I do to prepare for it?

It is perfectly normal to feel anxious prior to your surgery. In usual situations we advise people not to make decisions when they are under stress or to wait 6 months following a stressful event. In this situation, however, we are expecting you to receive bad news about your diagnosis, and to move quickly in making important life changing decisions undoubtedly at the most stressful time in your life. Your emotions, and those of the people around you, are certainly going to be difficult to manage and we suggest that you surround yourself with individuals with a positive attitude who will be support-ive and caring.

There will be a series of tests to evaluate you for sur-gery, as we have previously outlined. It is important that you keep all of your scheduled appointments, as you do not want to risk having your surgery delayed. If you are interested in having your blood banked, and if family members wish to donate blood directed to you for the day of surgery, you must make these arrangements as quickly as possible, as the process can be tedious and there is a prescribed amount of blood that one can donate and a specific timeframe in relation to your sur-gery. Donated blood also has a prescribed shelf life so call a local red cross collection center or the blood bank at the hospital where the surgery is to be performed in order to get the necessary details as soon as you have decided that you may have an interest in blood banking.

Continue to exercise if you have been doing so; if not, try to incorporate some light exercise to your daily rou-tine, even if this entails just a short walk a few times per day. It is difficult to maintain your weight follow-ing surgery so now is *not* the time to try to lose weight (unless you are obese and have been advised to do so). A diet rich in protein and high in calories is best followed as much as possible both prior to, and after, surgery. If you are having difficulty keeping up with your current weight, schedule an appointment with a dietician to get advice on how to best optimize your nutritional status.

Keep a list of all of your medications, both those that are prescribed and over-the-counter medications. Many seemingly harmless drugs and even nutritional supple-ments can have an effect on your ability to stop bleed-ing, which can obviously cause serious problems during and after surgery. Your doctors will advise you as to which drugs and supplements you can safely take, and whether or when to discontinue some or all of them prior to surgery and when you can safely resume these various medications.

It is standard to have some routine tests a few days before surgery. This usually includes an EKG, a chest X-ray, and some blood work. You will also meet with the anesthesiologist, who is the doctor responsible for administering the medications that will put you to sleep during the operation. If you have had surgery in the past and have encountered any problems with regard to the administration of the anesthesia or pain control, now is the time to discuss them so that these issues can be avoided.

Smoking has a tremendously bad effect on surgical outcome and recovery. If you smoke, quit now!!!! If you think it will be helpful in allowing you to stop smoking more easily, we can prescribe medication that will help ease the discomfort of sudden smoking cessation.

If you drink alcohol on a regular basis, you must let the surgeon know. We need to plan in advance a method for reducing your dependence upon alcohol, as this too can cause serious difficulties during the recovery phase. Remember your surgeon is not here to judge your lifestyle choices but to ensure the best possible outcome from your surgery.

48. What tests will I need before surgery to define what procedure I can tolerate?

The surgeries performed for mesothelioma are not considered to be minor procedures. Even if you do not have a cardiac history, we will order a full cardiovascular workup. A **cardiologist** will evaluate you to see if your heart can withstand the rigors of this surgery. This doctor will be responsible for letting the surgeon know that, from a cardiac standpoint, you are fit for surgery. You will most likely undergo an **echocardiogram**, which evaluates how effectively your heart pumps blood. Depending on your past medical history or cardiac exam, further testing, such as a stress test, might be required. This is another illustration of how your medical team evaluates the risks and the benefits when planning for surgery.

We may plan on performing a PD but we always prepare for an EPP. Your right lung normally contributes 55% of pulmonary function and the left lung 45%. Before knowing whether a patient is a candidate for an EPP, it is a good idea to inform him or her what to expect if an entire lung may be removed. A pulmonary function test and a **quantitative lung perfusion scan** are routinely used to determine whether an individual is likely to be able to function adequately following the removal of a lung, based on the degree to which your pulmonary function is affected by the tumor and other preexisting lung disease. The perfusion scan assigns numbers to regions of the lung so that the surgeon can estimate the residual amount of lung function that will be left after the operation. This will enable a determination as to whether you require supplemental oxygen following the surgery and how long this may be required before your

Cardiologist

A specialist in the treatment of conditions related to the heart who performs the appropriate tests to see if a patient is functionally able to tolerate surgery for mesothelioma.

Echocardiogram

A test that uses sound waves to create a moving picture of the heart. The picture is much more detailed than an X-ray image and involves no radiation exposure.

Quantitative lung perfusion scan

A radioactive nuclear scan that allows the measurement of the function of individual lung segments that can be used to determine how an individual will tolerate loss of lung function for an operation for mesothelioma.

remaining lung is able to compensate for the lost tissue. More importantly, a relatively accurate determination is possible that will indicate your ability to return to a normal functional status without the need for ongoing permanent supplemental oxygen. These are all very important considerations that may determine whether or not you are able (or want!) to have surgery.

49. What should I expect following my surgery? What are the common complications of surgery for mesothelioma?

Whether you have a PD or an EPP, both are major endeavors. Recovery time will vary with each individual, but the average time it takes to regain your strength and energy is usually 4 to 6 weeks. Unfortunately, there is always some pain and discomfort after surgery. At the majority of centers performing these operations, patients receive an **epidural catheter** that is put in at the time of the operation. This catheter is inserted into the spine while you are asleep, and numbing medication is put into the catheter. This medication puts the whole chest to sleep temporarily after the operation. You can then cough and breathe deeply, without the severe pain from the extensive incision in the chest wall required to remove the lung, thus decreasing the chance of infection and other complications. The epidural catheter usually is kept in place for 3 days and is then removed. After it is removed, you will be switched to an oral (by mouth) narcotic pain medication, which again is aimed at controlling your pain to enable you to breathe as deeply as possible. Breathing deeply prevents parts of your remaining lung from collapsing, which would lead to

Epidural catheter

A catheter that allows injection of an anesthetic drug into the space between the wall of the spinal canal and the covering of the spinal cord. This is the most reliable means for short-term pain relief after an operation for mesothelioma.

accumulation of fluid and possibly pneumonia. Purposefully forcing yourself to take deep breaths and practicing this before the operation is a good idea to optimize your recovery. Some institutions will arrange for you to get chest physical therapy aimed at forcing you to breathe as deeply as possible, at least for limited periods of the day, but concentrating on this yourself during as much of the recovery period as you can will certainly facilitate your recovery with less likelihood for a serious hospital-acquired pneumonia. You will continue to take this pain medication even after you are discharged and sent home. Gradually, over the next few weeks, your need for pain medications will decrease and you may be weaned off the narcotics and onto other forms of pain medicine that are not as strong, or you may not need to take any pain medication at all. It is important during this postoperative period that you communicate clearly the status of your pain with your medical attendants, especially in the early recovery period, so that you are neither too drowsy nor in too much pain to take deep breaths as this has such an important impact on both the rapidity and safety of your recovery period

Chest tubes are also inserted during surgery. These small, flexible tubes will be present when you awake and will remain in place until the lung has healed and there is a marginal amount of fluid coming from the chest. The purpose of the tubes is to drain fluid and air that have naturally collected in the chest cavity due to and during the surgery.

You may feel short of breath after surgery and could require oxygen temporarily. Breathing does improve over time, and the need for oxygen will also decrease as you get further out from the surgery. Many patients find that they benefit from pulmonary rehabilitation, which you can do at a center close to your home. It is usually covered on a one-time basis by your insurance, but you can contract with them to pay out of pocket should the need arise again in the future for you to undergo this form of physical therapy. Exercise, mild to moderate in intensity, can benefit you once you have completed the acute postoperative recovery course and will have an impact on the overall recovery of your pulmonary function.

When PDs are performed routinely for mesothelioma, few major complications are usually seen. Allowing the lungs to heal after stripping the pleura may require the chest tubes to remain in the chest cavity for longer than usual, sometimes up to 10 days. Pneumonia and respiratory problems can occur and are usually related to the size of the mass removed and the degree of presurgical decreased level of functioning. **Empyema** (the accumulation of pus in the chest) is rare and is managed by a more prolonged period of chest tube drainage together with **intravenous (IV)** and/or oral antibiotics. **Hemorrhage** or bleeding, that is severe enough to require the surgeon to re-open the chest cavity to find the cause and correct it, is very rare. Again, breathing deeply as much as you are able to as soon as you are able to after the surgery can impact the rate and degree of your recovery and again, a careful titration of pain medications is important so that you can comfortably achieve this goal without too much pain.

Due to the size and magnitude of the operation, an EPP has more risk of complications than a PD. The most common complication is an **arrhythmia** (abnormal heart beat), usually one that is fast and irregular. These occur because the heart is being manipulated during surgery and becomes irritated. The treatment for an arrhythmia involves starting the patient on specific

Empyema

Infected fluid (pus) in the chest that can result postoperatively as a complication of surgery for mesothelioma.

Intravenous (IV)

Within a blood vessel.

Hemorrhage

In medicine, loss of blood from damaged blood vessels. A hemorrhage may be internal or external, and usually involves a lot of bleeding in a short time.

Arrhythmia

Any deviation from or disturbance of the normal heart rhythm.

medications. Patients are usually kept on these medications by mouth for about 1 month after surgery, and then they can be stopped as long as the rhythm has been corrected. The most feared complication after an EPP is when the main bronchus (tube through which the air travels to each lung) to the lung that has been removed, develops an opening, allowing air to escape into the empty chest cavity. Fluid also drains through this hole, further filling the empty cavity or extending across to the normal lung cavity, thus further compromising breathing. This is known as a **broncho-pleural fistula** and may require a second operation to repair the opening, or external drainage with later repair if the problem occurs at some time after the original operation. The most common symptom of a broncho-pleural fistula is a persistent cough, so if a cough develops, make sure to inform your surgeon of its occurrence so that he can assess its cause. This complication can lead to pulmonary failure, pneumonia, and death. Recognized early, however, it can be treated successfully.

A heart attack as well as a clot going to the remaining lung from the legs (deep vein thrombosis and a **pulmonary embolism**) are also significant risks after an EPP, the latter due to the more prolonged period of bed rest. Finally, rare but dramatic complications can include the heart falling through an opening in the newly constructed pericardium (hernia), or failure of the newly constructed diaphragm to keep the abdominal contents out of the chest (chiefly on the left side). These reconstructions are performed with foreign material, usually some type of mesh, and there is a remote chance that they can become infected and need to be removed. Rapid accumulation of fluid in the chest once you start eating, or a change in the color of the chest tube drainage to a grayish, puss color could mean that the tube

Broncho-pleural fistula

A complication after extrapleural pneumonectomy in which there is a leakage of air from the closed bronchial tube.

Pulmonary embolism

Migration of a clot, usually from the legs, to the heart resulting in the blockage of arteries to the lung and resulting in acute shortness of breath. A possible cause of morbidity and mortality from operations for mesothelioma.

carrying lymph from the belly through the chest has been injured. In cases of EPPs, this situation may call for a second operation to close the leak, while with PDs, continued drainage and changing the patient's diet (decreasing the amount of fat in the diet) may allow this to close spontaneously.

Sarah adds . . .

Phil's recovery from surgery was relatively complication free. He went home 6 days after his surgery and was taking brief walks near our home within 2 weeks. A few weeks later, he returned to work. He was cautious about not overextending himself but was grateful to return to a daily routine that provided a distraction from the diagnosis.

50. What is chemotherapy? How does it work?

Chemotherapy is a general term to describe the use of chemicals or medications to treat disease, especially cancer. It's the treatment of cancer with a special group of drugs that are able to destroy cancer cells. There are many types of chemotherapy drugs, and each has a different way of attacking the cancer cells. In cancer treatment these medications can be used alone, but are more often used in various combinations to get the best overall effect. Studies have shown that these drugs work better when they are used with other types of chemotherapy agents than they do when given by themselves. Chemotherapy is considered the systemic treatment for mesothelioma because it is able to go to most parts of the body through the bloodstream. This means that chemotherapy is able to travel through the body, looking for any cancer cells that may have broken away from the original tumor.

Normal cells in the body grow and then die in a very precise and controlled fashion. Cancer cells, however, continue to grow, divide, and multiply uncontrollably. Chemotherapy interferes with this growth and stops cancer cells from reproducing at certain points in their life cycle. This, in turn, kills these cancer cells, but at the same time, it also affects a percentage of normal cells. The reason that this happens is that anticancer drugs act on any cells in the body that are dividing, not just cancer cells. The reason why more cancer cells are killed than normal cells is because the more rapidly dividing cells are preferentially killed by these drugs. However, there are relatively rapidly dividing normal cells that are more significantly affected than other normal cells, and these are the areas where most complications from chemotherapy are experienced. This is the cause of many of the side effects that are commonly seen during chemotherapy treatment. The types of cells that are most likely to be affected include those in the gastrointestinal (GI) tract (mouth pain, ulcers, diarrhea, bleeding), bone marrow (decrease in white cells, platelets, and/or red cells, and thus the increased risk for infection, bleeding, and/or anemia), hair follicles, (hair loss) and reproductive system (sterility).

Chemotherapy can be given by itself as the primary treatment to help keep the cancer from spreading, to shrink the tumor, or to relieve symptoms. It may also cure cancer in some types of tumors. It is more common, however, to see chemotherapy combined with other forms of treatment like surgery and radiation. In some instances, chemotherapy can be used before surgery to help shrink the tumor and make the surgery easier to perform (neo-adjuvant chemotherapy). It may also be used after surgery to help get rid of any cancer cells that may be left behind and that are too small to have been

TREATMENT

seen. When chemotherapy is used in this way it is called **adjuvant chemotherapy**.

Adjuvant chemotherapy

Treatment given after the primary treatment to increase the chances of a cure. Adjuvant therapy may include chemotherapy, radiation therapy, hormone therapy, or biological therapy.

51. What can I expect during chemotherapy? How many treatments will I need?

Your doctor will decide which chemotherapy drugs you will receive. Chemotherapy can be given in a number of places, and the choice depends on the types of drugs ordered, the policies of the hospital, and what your doctor prefers. It can be given in a clinic, in your hospital's outpatient department, or in a hospital. If you receive chemotherapy in the hospital, you may have to stay overnight so that the doctor can watch you closely. He or she will watch you for any side effects that might occur from the medications you receive and make changes as necessary. Chemotherapy drugs can be given by mouth, through a vein, or directly into an organ or body cavity. Some insurance companies pay for chemotherapy if it is administered in particular locations. They may not pay for chemotherapy in an independent facility, but might do so in a hospital outpatient chemotherapy suite. Many pharmaceutical companies have special programs for those that cannot afford their drugs or have very high insurance deductibles. If you are anticipating such issues, you may want to be in touch with a social worker associated with your doctor's office, as they can often help direct you either to the appropriate state or federal agencies or to drug company Web sites where you can download the forms necessary to apply for assistance with drug payments or free drugs.

The chemotherapy you will receive will most likely be administered directly into your vein (IV) through a thin needle or catheter that allows the drug to enter directly into your bloodstream. Having the needle placed for an IV feels the same as having blood drawn from a vein for a blood test. The difference is that during the chemotherapy administration, the needle remains in place for a longer period of time. Sometimes you may feel a cool sensation or slight burning at the insertion site when the IV is started. If you notice any burning, pain, or discomfort during or after an IV treatment, let your nurse or doctor know right away. Some drugs may cause redness and damage to the tissue if they leak out of the vein. A more permanent type of catheter may be necessary if a person has any type of problem with access to their veins or if it becomes difficult to insert the needle into a vein for each treatment. A doctor will insert this catheter into a large vein, and it will remain in place throughout your whole course of treatment. There are different types of catheters that are used for this purpose. Some are implanted under the skin and thus require little care, other than flushing, to prevent them from blocking up once the incision has healed, but these catheters are obviously harder to remove in that they require a second minor surgical procedure to do so. Other catheters extend through the skin, are relatively easily inserted and removed when treatment is completed, but there is a higher risk of infection at the skin entry site if you do not take proper care of the catheter. On the other hand, if properly cared for, these catheters can remain in place for many months during which time all blood draws, chemotherapy, fluids, and potential blood transfusions can be administered through them. Your doctor will explain to you which catheter he or she is recommending having placed and what you need to do to take care of it. Certainly, again, this is an issue in which your preference is an important consideration. You need to be as informed as possible about each type so as to make the best decision as to which one to request, unless there is a particular medical reason why one type is preferred over the other.

In peritoneal mesothelioma, the standard of care has been to perform a debulking procedure (removal of as much visible disease as is possible) and then to administer the chemotherapy directly into your abdomen at the time of surgery. This is referred to as HIPEC. The side effects are quite different from systemic chemotherapy and you will need some assistance in identifying which centers do this procedure and have a surgeon who has a true interest in mesothelioma. This is another instance where the Meso Foundation can assist you in identifying the right expert.

You should always let your doctor know what medications you are taking before you start treatment. Some medications should not be taken while you are receiving chemotherapy because they can interfere with the effects of the drug. Remember to report even over-the-counter drugs like vitamins and cold pills. Your doctor will let you know if you should stop taking any of them. After your treatment begins, let your doctor know of any changes in your medications, and check with him or her before starting anything new, including supplements or complementary medical drugs.

Your doctor will decide how many treatments of chemotherapy you will receive, the specific doses, and how often they will be given. The choice depends on the drugs that are being used and how your body responds to them. You may receive treatment every day, once a week, or every few weeks. It is often given with rest periods in between doses so that your body has a chance to recover from the effects of treatment and build healthy new cells. This break also helps you to regain some strength before beginning the next chemotherapy cycle or session. The chemotherapy schedule is typically outlined in cycles (one treatment). A course of chemotherapy encompasses all the cycles in your entire treatment plan. Cycle lengths can vary, but a typical chemotherapy course consists of multiple cycles of chemotherapy separated by some rest periods. In most cases you will receive approximately two or three cycles of the drugs and then be re-evaluated with CT scans to see if your cancer is responding to the treatment. The doctor will then decide what the next step in the plan will be. It is important to follow the schedule that your doctor lays out for you so that you can receive the desired effect from the chemotherapy. If you miss, or are unable to make a treatment session, contact your doctor immediately so that you can receive instructions about what to do.

52. Why are blood tests ordered during my chemotherapy treatment? What are blood counts, and what should I know about them?

Cancer cells grow and divide rapidly, and chemotherapy drugs are aimed at killing these types of cells. Unfortunately, they also harm healthy cells that divide rapidly. There are three major types of blood cells in the blood, all of which are made in the bone marrow. As with all cells in the body, each blood cell has a specific function and normal life span, so they are constantly being replaced by new cells made in the bone marrow. A common side effect of chemotherapy is that it damages healthy bone marrow cells, and causes a temporary shortage of the healthy cells. The three major types of blood cells include white blood cells (cells that help to fight infection), red blood cells (cells that carry oxygen to all parts of the body), and platelets (cells that cause the blood to clot). A blood test (CBC) will be ordered each week to check the levels of each of these blood cells, to make sure they are at an acceptable level in the bloodstream.

Chemotherapy can drastically lower the number of white blood cells that are available to help your body fight off infection. Your risk of getting an infection is much higher when these cells are low. Infections can occur in almost any part of the body, but most commonly affect the lungs, urinary tract, skin around the anus and rectum, and mouth. If your white blood cell count (WCC) falls too low, your doctor may decide to delay your next treatment, prescribe medication that can help your bone marrow make new white blood cells, or give you a lower dose of chemotherapy to give these cells a chance to recover. You may also, if your WCC drops below 1,000, be placed on antibiotics that will help prevent or ameliorate any infection should you get one (this is know as prophylactic antibiotics).

Chemotherapy can also cause a decrease in the number of red blood cells, which deliver oxygen to the tissues in the body. If these cells are decreased, the tissues may not be getting enough oxygen to do what they need to do. This is also known as anemia and can cause a person to feel extremely tired. It can also cause dizziness, shortness of breath, and feeling cold or weak. If your red blood cell count (hemoglobin, RBC) becomes too low, you might need medication that can help your bone marrow make new red blood cells or a blood transfusion. The number of platelets in your bloodstream could be decreased because of your treatment and its effect on the bone marrow. Platelets help stop bleeding by causing the blood to clot. You may notice that you bleed or bruise more easily when your platelets are low. If your platelet count becomes too low, your doctor may give you a transfusion of platelets. Because of the risk of low platelets during chemotherapy, it's important to notify your healthcare team if you notice any bleeding from the nose or the gums, red spots on the skin, unexpected bruising, or bloody bowel movements.

Some drugs that are used to treat mesothelioma require optimal kidney function. Some drugs can deplete certain minerals from the body, including potassium, sodium, magnesium, and/or phosphate. A blood metabolic panel (either BMP or CMP) will be drawn together with the CBC to determine if it is safe to use a particular drug and to assess ongoing organ and electrolyte status as you proceed with the treatment. We often adjust drug doses, change drugs, or prescribe supplements to ensure that you can safely receive your chemotherapy.

It is thus *very* important that your doctor monitor these blood cell counts frequently by ordering a complete blood cell count (CBC) and platelet count as part of your routine blood work, as well as the more specialized blood testing as mentioned in the previous paragraph.

53. What are the common side effects of chemotherapy?

There are many side effects of chemotherapy that you might experience. You might know other people undergoing treatment or who have received treatment in the past. Unless they have had positive experiences with their treatment, tune them out. It is important to approach chemotherapy as a necessity that will help you be successful in battling your cancer. Each drug has a different side effect profile and prior to being administered, you should have had a full discussion with your doctor on what to expect during chemotherapy. Let's focus first on pemetrexed (Alimta) which, combined with cisplatin, is the only regimen approved by the Food and Drug Administration (FDA) for the treatment of mesothelioma. Hopefully, we will soon have other drugs approved so with that in mind, we will address more generalized side effects that may occur during treatment toward the later part of this question.

Pemetrexed is generally a well-tolerated drug. As mentioned earlier, chemotherapy can also have an impact on good cells that rapidly divide as well as malignant cells. The cells most affected are those that line the oral mucosa and GI tract. When these cells are adversely affected, we can experience a number of side effects. The most common side effect can be nausea/vomiting, which is generally well controlled with special medications called antiemetics. You should ask for prescriptions prior to the day of administration so that you can have them filled and waiting for you at home. Some might require prior authorization by your doctor's office staff in order to be available to you, so again, advanced planning will get this resolved in time for your treatment. Some patients have reported mouth sores, which can make eating and oral hygiene uncomfortable. Your doctor can prescribe a special mouthwash that will ease this discomfort. Some patients also benefit from mixing 1 tablespoon of baking soda into an 8-oz glass of water, which will neutralize acid in your mouth. Both of these interventions are very helpful, so please do inform your doctor if you begin to develop any sores or discomfort in your oral cavity. Some patients will develop diarrhea while on therapy while others become constipated, a problem that may be a side effect from some of the antinausea medications. Both of these symptoms can be unpleasant, and, again, we have medications that can help prevent these problems or ameliorate them if they occur. Make sure you inform your doctor or treating team at the earliest sign of a side effect so they can prescribe appropriate medications to control these side effects.

Cisplatin, which is most often given in conjunction with pemetrexed, can cause damage to your kidneys. You will be encouraged to drink additional fluids in the days before and following your therapy. You will also be given extra fluid in your IV to prevent this damage at the time that you receive the drug. Another common side effect of cisplatin is hearing loss. It is very important that you discuss any hearing difficulties you already have with your doctor prior to receiving on cisplatin. If you do notice changes during therapy, inform your doctor immediately, as they could indicate a necessary modification of your regimen. A final relatively common complication is peripheral nerve damage or a peripheral **neuropathy**. This causes a loss of feeling in the extremities, starting in the fingers and toes and advancing upwards if progressive. It can also be associated with tingling, changes in temperature sensation, and even mild-to-severe pain in the palms and or soles. Again, if you note such changes or think that they may be developing, you should discuss this with your treatment team so that an assessment can be made as to whether you should continue with the cisplatin or switch to an alternative drug. There is another drug, carboplatin, that is very similar to cisplatin and can sometimes be substituted or given as a replacement in patients who we think may not tolerate cisplatin or are developing side effects to cisplatin that are not as usual with the use of

Neuropathy

A problem in peripheral nerve function (any part of the nervous system except the brain and spinal cord) that causes pain, numbness, tingling, swelling, and muscle weakness in various parts of the body; also called peripheral neuropathy. Neuropathies can be caused by physical injury, infection, toxic substances, disease (such as cancer, diabetes, kidney failure, or malnutrition), or drugs such as anticancer drugs.

carboplatin. Carboplatin less commonly causes kidney damage, hearing loss, and neuropathy, but more significantly affects the bone marrow.

Most people have questions and concerns about the side effects of chemotherapy. It is often overwhelming to hear the wide range of possible side effects associated with these drugs. We are required to discuss most of the side effects associated with a particular drug, but you can also ask your oncologist which are the more common side effects that are reported so that you can concentrate more on what you might expect rather than on rare issues that you may never experience. In general, it is less frightening to incur a side effect that you have already been warned about than to have an effect that you were not expecting. As you can see from what we have already discussed, there are ways of dealing with most of the common side effects so that the ordeal need not be as daunting as is usually made out in the lay press/literature or by others who have undergone chemotherapy in the past.

There are a few side effects that are commonly seen in people receiving chemotherapy. Remember these are possible side effects (you may experience one or two or even none, but it is unlikely that you will experience all) and you should, as we have mentioned, discuss in detail which ones you might expect with your treatment team. These include fatigue, nausea, vomiting, and hair loss. Other effects that can occur include constipation, diarrhea, blood clots, decreased blood counts, and neuropathies (loss of sensation and/or tingling in the hands and feet). These occur because normal, rapidly growing cells in the digestive tract, reproductive system, bone marrow, and hair follicles can be damaged by anticancer drugs. Some side effects are minor and annoying, while others can be severe. If severe, they may prevent you from receiving your chemotherapy as the doctor originally planned, which might involve a delay in treatment or a change in that treatment. However, it is important to report any effects, even if that requires some change or delay in therapy, as the development of a severe complication can significantly compromise your quality of life so that whatever you gain from the chemotherapy can be negated by these negative, and sometimes permanent, effects. After you have received all of your chemotherapy and your normal cells have had a chance to recover, most of the side effects you experienced will gradually disappear. Some of them will go away quickly while others may take months. Occasionally, some can cause permanent damage. Side effects can be discouraging and bothersome, but they must be compared and weighed against the chemotherapy's ability to kill the cancer cells. Let your doctor or nurse know of any difficulties you are experiencing so he or she can offer suggestions on how to manage these side effects and how seriously they need to be viewed in terms of your ongoing treatment.

54. What is radiation therapy?

Radiation therapy is a type of cancer treatment that kills cancer cells by targeting their DNA. It can be given as part of a multimodality course of treatment before or after surgery, or it can be given as a single form of treatment. Usually in those circumstances, it is used to control some specific complication from a tumor mass, such as pain due to nerve impingement or organ failure due to a tumor that may be obstructing or infiltrating an important internal organ of the body.

Following surgery, radiation is often given to the original area of the tumor. In this situation, it is meant to prevent the tumor from recurring and does not target disease that has become systemic or spread beyond the original site of the disease. Radiation therapy can also be used in combination with other treatments, such as chemotherapy. This combination can enhance the effect of each of the therapies in being able to kill cancer cells both at the site of an original tumor mass and in attempting to kill all other cells, which may have broken away from the original tumor or which may be infiltrating (burrowing into) adjacent tissues or organs. Other names for radiation therapy include irradiation, radiotherapy, cobalt treatment, and X-ray therapy. Special cancer doctors, radiation oncologists, are responsible for providing this type of treatment. They will work with your doctor to decide on the type, amount, and frequency of your treatment with radiation. If you are to receive radiation therapy, you will have a meeting with the radiation oncologist beforehand to discuss the treatment plan.

55. How does radiation work?

Radiation therapy uses high-energy rays to kill cancer cells. Doctors first discovered that they could use radiation (X-rays) to help them see inside the human body and locate disease. Soon after, they discovered that these same rays could be used to treat disease as well. These rays are carefully directed at tumors for brief periods and cause the cancer cells to become injured. This prevents the cancer cells from growing and dividing, which in turn kills the cells and slows down or stops the growth of the tumor. Unfortunately, normal cells in the treatment area are also affected by this radiation, but are hopefully more able to recover or be replaced by other normal cells so that you do not experience any permanent side effects. Again, as with chemotherapy, radiation targets the more rapidly dividing cells so that depending where the radiation is targeted, similar side effects as with chemotherapy may be experienced. If in the neck region, the mouth, throat, and esophagus (swallowing tube) may be affected resulting in mouth sores, ulcers, pain, and difficulty eating that may last several days or weeks depending on the dose of radiation therapy given and the tolerance of a particular part of the body to that dose. One important aspect of radiation therapy is that there is a limited amount that can be given to a specific area as the effects on normal tissue is cumulative. All organs such as the lungs, liver, kidneys, bones, brain, spinal cord, and soft tissues have a specific threshold of radiation that they can be exposed to, after which permanent damage to that organ may occur. The bones, for example, can withstand much higher doses of radiation than the lungs can, making the amount that can be given to a particular spot in the chest, for example, limited by the potential for underlying lung damage. This would thus complicate the treatment of a mass in an individual who had previously lost one lung as a result of primary surgical treatment of an earlier pleural mesothelioma for whom new disease is now noted on or in the remaining healthy lung or chest cavity.

56. What is a dose of radiation, and how many treatments will I need?

The radiation treatment plan that is recommended for you will depend on the type of operation you have, your general health, your test results, and the other treatments you are receiving. After your initial meeting with the radiation oncologist and prior to actually beginning any treatment, you will undergo treatment planning or simulation. At this time, the radiation oncologist will decide the exact location of treatment, the total dose of radiation that you will need, and the number of treatments required. The total dose of radiation is divided into daily doses called fractionation. This is to ensure that it does its intended job with the least amount of damage to your normal cells. The number of radiation treatments required will vary depending on your individual situation, the site being irradiated, and the possibility that you may have received previous radiation to that area or nearby. Radiation treatments are usually given 5 days a week for several weeks but can also be given twice daily (hyperfractionation) for shorter periods or as a single dose.

This second visit to the radiation oncologist to undergo the simulation can take some hours, so it is important that you plan your day around this appointment. A radiation physicist or dosimetrist helps the radiation oncologist plan the treatment and is also responsible for making sure the treatment machines are functioning properly at all times. You will probably not receive a radiation treatment on this first visit, but will be given a daily radiation time and start date before you go home. At most of these visits to the radiation therapy department, it is not likely that you will see your radiation oncologist, but you will likely be treated by the same radiation technician (radiotherapist) each day who will be familiar with your specific needs and will convey to the radiation oncologist any concerns or side effects you may be experiencing. Usually you will see the radiation oncologist once a week or once every 2 weeks with a follow up visit 3–4 weeks after completing your radiation to discuss further follow-up and/or perhaps treatments. The maximal benefit from radiation is often only evident more than 6 weeks after completing the radiation, and it can take that period of time for all side effects, such as mouth pain, to disappear completely. You will of course not experience any mouth pain if the radiation beam is not directed at the mouth, the effects of radiation, as we have discussed, being entirely local. You may notice some reddening of the skin in the area that was radiated. This is much like a sunburn, and if painful, can be treated with topical lotions prescribed by the radiation therapists.

The exact place on the body where the high-energy rays will be directed is called the treatment area. A technologist will locate this area using an X-ray machine while you lie still on a table. After the area is located, the technologist or doctor will mark your skin with a colored indelible ink marker, creating a tattoo. This must not be washed off the skin until all your treatment has been completed. If for some reason the mark fades or comes off, do not try to draw it back on yourself. Instead, notify your doctor right away. Sometimes a plastic or plaster cast or form of the proposed treatment site has to be made. This form helps you to stay in the same position for each treatment and in some instances is also intended to shield normal areas, or more sensitive organs in the region to be treated, from excessive radiation exposure.

57. What equipment is used to deliver radiation?

The type of radiation you will probably receive is called **external beam radiation**. There are various machines that deliver this kind of radiation to the cancer,

External beam radiation

Radiation therapy that uses a machine to aim high-energy rays at the cancer; also called external radiation. Most commonly used after removal of an entire lung for mesothelioma.

Cobalt machine

A radioactive machine using a form of the metal cobalt, which is used as a source of radiation to treat cancer.

Linear accelerator

A machine that creates high-energy radiation to treat cancer, using electricity to form a stream of fast-moving subatomic particles. Also called linear accelerator or a linac.

including the **cobalt machine** and **linear accelerator**. These machines give the same type of treatment but work in slightly different ways. This equipment is located in either a hospital or special treatment center, and radiation is usually given as an outpatient treatment. There are many new developments in the field of radiation therapy and the focus is to try to minimize the effects of radiation on healthy tissue, while maximizing the effects on cancer cells, much as we try with chemotherapy. We are using more precise methods of delivering radiation therapy to the sites that are involved with your mesothelioma so as to minimize other local tissue damage, for example, to an underlying normal lung. Use caution in choosing your radiation facility, as an experienced center can minimize some of the risks involved with this therapy.

58. What can I expect during radiation?

Your doctor will be monitoring your progress throughout your radiation treatment. Since radiation affects both cancer cells and normal cells, you will again be checked regularly for any side effects that may occur. Blood tests will be performed, usually weekly, and the results reviewed with you by your radiotherapist and/or radiation oncologist. Alert your doctor, nurse, or radiotherapist if you notice any side effects or anything that you consider unusual so that they can be managed before they become severe or your treatment plan can be adjusted. Some people are able to continue doing things that they normally do while undergoing radiation treatment. Others find that they need more rest than usual. Your body is using a lot of extra energy during this time, and you might require more sleep than you normally do.

Be sure to listen to your body and rest as often as necessary. If you are receiving external beam radiation, you are not radioactive, and therefore you don't have to limit your contact with others. You do need to avoid anyone with an infection, such as a cold or flu, because your resistance could be lowered while you are undergoing treatment. It is also important to eat well during this time to try to maintain your weight and nutritional status. Communicate with your doctor, nurse, or technologist, and don't be afraid to ask questions. They are more than willing to help you through your treatment and advise you as necessary.

59. What is the actual radiation procedure like?

When you arrive for your treatment, you will probably be asked to put on a hospital gown. You will then be brought to the treatment room, where you will be assisted onto the treatment table. The radiation therapy technologist will position you and adjust the machines so that everything lines up with the marks on your skin. Special lead shields can be used to protect your normal organs and tissues. They are placed between the machine and the part of your body they are trying to protect. It is very important that you stay as still as possible throughout the entire treatment, which will usually last only a few minutes. However in some individuals who are in pain, it may be hard to lie in what may be an uncomfortable position for any length of time. If this is an issue, you should discuss a plan with your doctors for you to be given some form of pain medication a short while before you undergo the radiation so as to enable you to tolerate this, albeit relatively short, period. Once everything is set up, the technologist will leave the room and turn on the machine. He or she will control the machine from a nearby room and monitor all activities at the same time. Remember, the technologist is able to watch you through a window or on a TV screen during the entire treatment, and you can talk with him or her at all times through a speaker that connects the two rooms. The treatment machines do make noises as they move around your body. They are trying to get at the cancer from different angles and are under the technologist's control at all times. The noise these machines make can sound much like a vacuum cleaner. You should not feel any discomfort at all from the treatment itself, and you will not see or hear the radiation just as with any normal X-ray or scan. If you have any fears, or are not feeling well during the treatment, let the technologist know immediately.

60. How long does each treatment take?

The actual time required to deliver the radiation itself is very short. It takes only about 1–5 minutes to receive the actual treatment dose, even though you can be in the treatment room for 15–20 minutes, getting into the correct position for the treatment to be properly administered. There is no restriction on food during treatment, but you will have to exercise caution while out in the sun, as you will be more susceptible to sunburns in the area being exposed to radiation. Wear protective clothing and be generous when applying sunblock if you are outdoors on sunny days. Do not apply any lotions to the irradiated area unless approved by your radiation therapist, as some ingredients of these lotions may either enhance or detract from the radiation efficacy. Your skin might be particularly sensitive during treatment and the radiation center can recommend salves and lotions that will not interfere in any way with the administration of the therapy. Delays can happen at any point along the way, so it is important to remember that there may be times when you will have to wait longer than expected for your treatment. Your treatment time is negotiated before treatment starts and usually remains the same throughout your therapy. The radiation team will work with you to develop the best appointment schedule to suit your needs, but please let them know if you are going to be late or miss an appointment. To ensure that you get the most benefit from your treatment, you must receive all ordered doses. Therefore, if you miss an appointment, you will have to make up each missed dose at the end of your therapy.

61. What are the common side effects of radiation?

During the course of destroying cancer cells, radiation also damages normal cells that are in the treatment area or field. The end result is the development of side effects. These side effects depend on the part of the body being treated, the dose given, and the size of the radiation field. Some people don't experience any negative effects from their treatment, while most others have very few side effects. If you develop a severe side effect from the radiation, your doctor may want to give you a break from your treatment for a short period. Certain side effects are common no matter what area of the body is being treated. These include fatigue, loss of appetite, and skin reactions or irritations. Other side effects are related to the specific area of the body that is in within the treatment field. When receiving radiation to the chest area, you may experience certain side effects, including **esophagitis** (swelling of the esophagus), fibrosis (the formation of scar tissue), **pneumonitis**

Esophagitis

Inflammation of the esophagus, which is the tube that carries food from the mouth to the stomach. This most frequently occurs in the setting of chest radiation after an operation for mesothelioma.

Pneumonitis

An inflammatory infection that occurs in the lung.

(radiation lung injury), sore throat, and loss of hair in the treated area. Although it can happen, nausea is not commonly seen when receiving chest radiation. Be sure to discuss these specific side effects with your doctor or nurse and report any that occur. He or she will be able to help you deal with them and suggest ways to ameliorate the effects, which will resolve over the course of a few days to weeks after you complete the radiation therapy.

Remember, as before, that your medical or surgical oncologist is likely the primary coordinator of all your treatment, so if you have any concerns about the status of your disease and nature of your treatments, this is the person to speak to. Because the coordination of your therapy is so important, the need for you to have someone who is completely familiar with your problems in your doctor's office is very important, as that person will, in many ways, be your primary contact to all your treating physicians, whether that is your surgeon, medical oncologist, or radiation oncologist, or even some additional physician such as a cardiologist, pulmonologist, or gastroenterologist. All of these additional doctors will play a role in helping to maintain and improve your health, maintain your quality of life, and prolong your life, but your medical or surgical oncologist needs to be the person who guides and directs you through this very complicated maze of therapies. This is because their training is more encompassing of understanding the problems and needs of cancer patients through all phases of treatment from diagnosis to palliative and hospice care. This is, of course, another extremely compelling reason why it is so important to find an individual who is not only an expert on mesothelioma, but whom you can trust and who either makes him- or herself available to you at all times or has staff who can fulfill that role and liaise between you and your primary and other doctors. For many individuals who live far from where their primary therapy is administered, your local internist can likely assume some of that coordinating role, but he or she needs to understand that they need to be in close contact with the office of your primary treating oncologist so that there are no misunderstandings in terms of your treatment plans, follow-up needs, blood testing, and radiological studies to assess both your general health status as well as the status of your mesothelioma. Here again, you, or your primary caregiver if you cannot take charge yourself, need to be very proactive in playing a key role in making sure that things *do not* fall between the cracks. Maintaining a positive attitude, and being actively engaged and proactive in your care, are the best ways of you helping yourself in this fight against your mesothelioma! This includes maintaining your nutrition, exercising as much as you are able to, and being vigilant about issues relating to either treatment side effects or effects of your mesothelioma.

PART SIX

Decision Making

What are clinical trials?

What are some experimental or investigational treatments for mesothelioma?

How do I decide on a treatment plan when faced with multiple options?

More...

62. What are the standard treatment options for mesothelioma?

Chemotherapy has been used over the years to try to shrink these tumors. However, the problem with the older chemotherapy drugs is that they haven't worked very well. Doctors have now found that it may be best to combine surgery and chemotherapy, using newer drugs in people who are healthy enough to tolerate them. These newer drugs have been found to work better than the drugs used in the past, and combining them with surgery could allow people to live longer.

First line (the first chemotherapy treatment used to treat your cancer) chemotherapy regimen for mesothelioma is generally a combination of two chemotherapeutic agents, cisplatin and pemetrexed. Cisplatin is an alkylating agent (a drug that works by attaching an alkyl agent to the DNA of cells, the theory being that cancer cells are destroyed through this process). Cisplatin is administered by IV, and there is no oral form. Since cisplatin is an irritant (can cause inflammation of the veins), it is very important to let your doctor or nurse know if you experience any discomfort at the IV site during or after the infusion. The dose of the drug will depend on many factors including your age, height, weight, and general health status, particularly your kidney function. Cisplatin is given over 1–2 hours every 3 weeks.

Cisplatin affects normal cells just like all other chemotherapies, so possible side effects include low blood cell counts as well as fatigue, nausea, and hair loss, as discussed earlier. There are some specific side effects of cisplatin. The drug can cause damage to the kidneys. For this reason, your doctor will check your baseline kidney

First-line therapy

Refers to the first treatment you receive for your mesothelioma diagnosis. Alimta and cisplatin are the only first-line treatments approved in the United States for the treatment of malignant mesothelioma.

function (labs to measure kidney function) before you receive any cisplatin to determine if your kidneys are functioning well enough to process the drug. While you're on cisplatin therapy, there are some actions that can be taken to reduce the risk of kidney damage, such as giving you extra intravenous fluid hydration, and encouraging you to increase the fluids that you drink. This extra fluid helps to quickly flush the medicine out of your system by increasing your kidney function and ultimately protect your kidneys. Because of the intravenous fluids before and after cisplatin, the total infusion time might take up to 5 hours.

Cisplatin can also change the taste of certain foods, and may cause a metallic taste in your mouth. Peripheral neuropathy is a side effect of cisplatin that affects the nervous system and can cause numbness, tingling, burning, pain, or weakness in your hands and/or feet. There are some medications that can ameliorate the pain of neuropathy if it develops. There is a rare chance that cisplatin can affect hearing and your inner ear. Let your doctor know immediately if you notice any hearing changes or ringing in your ears.

Cisplatin should be given once in a 21-day cycle (every 3 weeks), in combination with pemetrexed. Your doctor will likely want to see you in between treatments. They will look at certain blood values, such as the CBC (a simple blood test that calculates the concentration of white blood cells, red blood cells, and platelets in the blood). They might also draw a chemistry panel, which looks at the measures of kidney and liver function and electrolytes (the minerals that help keep the body's fluid levels in balance and are necessary to help the muscles, heart, and other organs working properly).

DECISION MAKING

Alimta (pemetrexed)

Pemetrexed is a relatively new chemotherapy drug. Following years of clinical trials, it was approved by the FDA in 2004. Pemetrexed can be given alone, but is more commonly given in combination with cisplatin. It works by interfering with enzymes (proteins that speed up chemical reactions) that the cancer cell needs to replicate. It blocks folate (all cells use B-vitamins, such as folate, to make new genetic material), thus by blocking the folate pathway in cancer cells, which disrupts the cells' ability to grow and replicate. To lower the chances of side effects with pemetrexed, it is necessary to take folic acid and vitamin B12 before, during, and after treatment. Your doctor will prescribe a folic acid tablet for at least 5–7 days before you start pemetrexed. If you are already taking a multivitamin, it probably contains 400–800 mcg of folic acid; this is the correct dose and any additional folic acid may alter the effectiveness of pemetrexed. Inform your medical team if you are taking a multivitamin as you most likely will not require additional folic acid. You will continue taking the folic acid every day until 21 days after your last cycle of pemetrexed. You will need a B-12 injection within the week before you start the pemetrexed. B-12 injections will be given about every 9 weeks while you are on this chemotherapy.

Common side effects of pemetrexed include decreased blood counts, fatigue, and nausea and vomiting. Skin reactions including rash can also occur so it's important to let your doctor know if you notice any rash during or after you receive pemetrexed. Your doctor may prescribe a steroid tablet for you to take twice daily the day before, the day of, and the day after the chemotherapy infusion to lessen the likelihood of skin reactions. Pemetrexed is also associated with a decreased appetite and diarrhea. If the diarrhea or vomiting becomes too severe, this can cause dehydration (losing more fluid than you take in, so your body becomes so fluid-depleted that it doesn't have enough water to carry out normal function). Mouth sores (stomatitis) can also occur, and you should let your doctor know if they develop so that they can be treated immediately.

Pemetrexed is given as an intravenous infusion once in a 21-day cycle (every 3 weeks). The infusion runs over 10 minutes. The dose of the drug will depend on many factors including your age, height, weight, and general health status. Your doctor may see you between treatment doses while you're taking Pemetrexed to examine you and draw a CBC in order to make sure the drug has not caused your blood cell counts to drop too low.

Following treatment with pemetrexed and cisplatin, you may have a respite period until your tumor begins to, once again, become active. This is the time to explore **second-line therapy**. There are many drugs and combinations of drugs that have demonstrated some activity in mesothelioma but have not been studied in large enough numbers to get FDA designation as approved second-line therapy specifically for mesothelioma.

Second-line therapy

Therapy that is introduced if a patient has failed to respond or is no longer tolerating the initial treatment.

Insurance companies can deny these therapies but in many cases, will permit treatment once a denial followed by an appeal process takes place. Each insurance plan is different, but getting approval for the off-label use of a drug, approved for use in cancers other than mesothelioma, is an often lengthy multistep process that takes several weeks, thus creating much anxiety and angst. In most cases, this process is resolved successfully and permission is granted for you to receive the drug in question. There are, however, instances in which the drug is persistently denied, in which case you and your doctor may have to discuss either the use of an alternative agent or alternative strategies for you to obtain the drug. These strategies may include: (1) getting legal advice and support; (2) paying out of pocket for a drug, which may be extremely costly; or (3) trying to get support from some foundation or perhaps the drug company that makes the drug in order to pay a more nominal amount for the drug If you have completed your initial treatment and are in the "watch-and-wait" phase, you have the time to explore these potential second-line therapies or next treatment options. There are usually a number of clinical trials available for such second-line therapies, but there are factors that make you eligible or ineligible for these trials. Second-line therapies that are not part of a trial can be used at any time, but clinical studies usually require that you have failed one standard regimen and sometimes will disqualify you if you have had additional treatments so it is important to get this right and leave as many options open as possible for future needs. If your tumor has progressed and you need to seek immediate treatment, understand that a new treatment will not be initiated until you are at least 4 or more weeks out from having completed your last treatment. This interval is important in that we want any toxicities from the prior regimen to have completely resolved so there will be no confusion as to whether side effects you subsequently develop are due to the original drugs or the new ones that have been introduced. You will also need a new complete workup of the nature and extent of your disease, which usually will include laboratory and radiological studies. If you are entered on a protocol, you might additionally require some protocol-specific testing.

Scans are planned close to the time of the start of your new regimen so measurements can be obtained of your residual or new tumors for accurate future comparison. If you have been entered into a clinical trial with a new agent not yet approved for mesothelioma or any other cancer, you will be given the drug at no cost, but will incur costs associated with what is considered the standard of care, including laboratory studies or other evaluations that would normally be done even if you were not entered on a clinical study. This should all be discussed with you at the time of the consent process. You have a right to know your financial obligations and should insist upon and receive a full disclosure of what to expect. If you are having financial difficulties, then you should schedule an appointment with a social worker. They are trained to discuss and help you resolve insurance issues, help you identify organizations that provide financial assistance, and network with pharmaceutical companies to help you obtain free or discounted drugs. This is a valuable resource, as is the case manager assigned to you by your insurance plan.

The role of radiation in mesothelioma has really been undefined. It has been used to try to control symptoms associated with cancer, such as pain. However, it has not been found to be of benefit as a primary treatment option. Radiation therapy is now being used as part of a combination package with surgery or with surgery and chemotherapy to assess whether it can kill the cancer cells remaining after surgery and prevent the cancer from coming back, particularly in the setting of mesothelioma that originates in the chest. There is much research that still needs to be done in this field, and clinical trials are currently underway that are trying to answer these and other questions in order to find the best treatment options for people with mesothelioma both at the time of its original diagnosis as well as at times of **recurrence**.

Recurrence

The return of cancer after the tumor had disappeared at the same site as the original (primary) tumor or in another location.

63. *What are clinical trials?*

Clinical trials are medical research studies that are designed to evaluate new cancer treatments and the effects these treatments have on patients. They are one of the most important ways doctors have to improve care and move forward in the fight against cancer. They are designed to answer specific questions and give information on the safest and most effective ways to treat cancer. Patients who participate in these trials not only make contributions to science but also are able to receive new treatments before they are made available to the general public. The FDA oversees these clinical trials, which test certain promising drugs before they are approved for regular use. All experimental protocols must be thoroughly evaluated by the IRB of the hospital or institution where the study is to be conducted before any patient can be entered into that clinical trial.

Phase I trial

A study to understand how a drug works and what dose is best tolerated in human subjects. Safety of drug dosing is the main goal of this particular phase.

Phase II trial

A study to determine if a particular drug is effective in your cancer and to monitor and record any side effects associated with the drug.

Clinical trials have three different steps or phases. The earliest studies of a particular drug are called **phase I trials**. The goal of these early studies is to find out the safest and most appropriate dose that should be given and to identify the side effects most likely to be encountered in treating patients with the specific new drug. The treatment is offered only to patients who have not responded to standard treatments and have widespread disease, and especially to individuals who have failed all other standard and approved drugs. In other words, there is likely not much known about the efficacy of this treatment at this point and there may be a higher risk of side effects, so these treatments are offered to only a small number of patients in a very tightly controlled setting.

In a **phase II trial**, the new treatment has been found to have some anticancer activity and is being used to treat a particular type of cancer to see how well it works and to obtain more information about its overall effectiveness as well as its more general side effects. **Phase III trials** are used to compare a new treatment with the current, standard treatment that has already been proven effective for that type of cancer. In this type of study, doctors are trying to find out whether the new treatment is better than, equal to, or inferior to the established current therapy. These types of trials have two or more treatment arms that are being compared. A patient is randomized (assigned by chance, not by choice) to a particular treatment arm or group in the study and it is important that you realize that neither you nor your doctor can influence the decision as to which treatment arm you may be assigned to.

It is always the patient's decision to enter into a clinical trial. You will never be entered onto a study without your written consent.

Phase III trial
A study to test the drug against the standard of care to see how it measures up in comparison.

DECISION MAKING

64. How do I learn about clinical trials, and how do I decide whether a trial is right for me?

You can learn more about clinical trials by talking with your doctor or by contacting the Cancer Information Service of the National Cancer Institute. This is a free service that is available to you by dialing (800) 4-CANCER. Many different clinical trials are underway at institutions around the country. The Meso Foundation is a good source for information about the clinical trials options that are available throughout the country and can discuss with you which trials you can be eligible for based on your personal cancer and medical history. This can streamline the process and then you can consider requesting a second opinion to talk to other specialists about the trials they are conducting in their area.

Some people associate being in a clinical trial with being used as a guinea pig for experimentation. We would suggest that you look at this as an opportunity to try new treatments that would be unavailable to you unless you are in a clinical trial. Understanding what is involved with each trial and educating yourself as much as possible before making a decision will help to alleviate some of the fears and anxieties that go along with any clinical trial. Treatment decisions are often difficult to make; therefore it is important to discuss your options with the doctors involved in your care and with family members and others close to you. Although the final decision is yours to make, others should be able to help you think through your options. Write down a list of questions to ask your doctor so you don't forget something during your appointment.

There are certain things you should find out about the trial so that you know what it involves and what is required of you ahead of time. Asking questions may help you decide whether a trial is right for you and may also get rid of some of the uncertainties you have. Ask the doctor what the specific treatment is and what makes it different from the standard treatments. Also, find out about the specific side effects related to treatment. You will want to know how long the study will last, whether you have to be hospitalized for the treatment, and where the trial will take place. Lastly, cost is an important consideration for most people. Find out what your insurance will cover before you make your final decision about the trial. The cost of the drugs involved in these trials is usually covered by the study itself, but other expenses may not be covered. You will probably receive more tests and examinations by your doctor when you are in a clinical trial than you would normally receive. This is because your condition and progress must be closely monitored, and study data must be collected at specific intervals along the way. This monitoring is accomplished by following a carefully designed treatment plan called a protocol that spells out what will be done, when, and why.

If you do decide to participate in a clinical trial, you will be given an **informed consent** form to read over and sign before you are enrolled in the study. The informed consent entails much more than simply obtaining a signature on a form. The key to informed consent is education, as the informed consent serves to reinforce the information given to you by your physician regarding the drugs and other specific issues involved in the study. The consent document serves to fully explain, in lay terms, the information given to you by your physician regarding the trial including its potential risks and benefits. Signing the consent means that you have received information about the trial and that you are freely agreeing to be a part of the study. Remember that it is a personal choice to enroll in a study, and therefore you can always refuse to be a part of any clinical trial. Also keep in mind that you may withdraw from a study at any time along the way for any reason and that there may also be circumstances in which your physician or the sponsor of the study may feel it is appropriate to remove you prematurely from the study. All of these possibilities are usually described and discussed in the consent document.

Informed consent

A process in which a person learns key facts about a clinical trial including potential risks and benefits before deciding whether or not to participate in a study. Informed consent continues throughout the trial.

DECISION MAKING

111

65. What if I don't qualify for a clinical trial?

All clinical trials have eligibility criteria that patients must meet in order to participate. Many factors come into play in determining whether or not a person is eligible for a particular clinical trial. If you don't meet all the criteria, you will not be able to participate in that trial. This means that specific characteristics of your health or cancer don't match with the study and its requirements. However, this does not mean that you are ineligible for other clinical trials and that at some future time, you may fit the eligibility criteria of that study. If you do not fit into any clinical trial at this time, other treatment options may be available to you that are still considered among the standard treatments for your mesothelioma.

66. What are some experimental or investigational treatments for mesothelioma?

There is a growing interest in mesothelioma research and many new therapies are being investigated. Biologic therapy, which is today a commonly encountered term in clinical trials of cancer, involves the use of agents derived from biologic sources and/or affecting biologic responses. These treatments are also referred to as biotherapy or immunotherapy. This would include some of the new vaccine trials that are currently available following first-line therapy or successful completion of your surgery and other possible treatments.

Monoclonal antibodies (MoAbs) are molecules/drugs artificially produced in a laboratory that are designed to bind to specific protein structures (antigens) expressed on the surface of malignant cells. These drugs are designed to block the growth of the tumor and/or recruit the body's immune system to attack the cancer cells. They are generally given alone or sometimes in combination with other therapies in a clinical trial. In the setting of mesothelioma, some of the new MoAbs under investigation target mesothelin, which is a protein found on the outside of epithelial mesothelioma cells. Mesothelin may additionally target other proteins that have been identified in malignant mesothelioma.

Gene therapy involves the use of DNA or RNA to change your individual genes in some way that is hoped to increase your body's ability to fight or prevent disease. There are a number of clinical trials underway using gene therapies as a means of controlling disease progression or enhancing the shrinkage of the tumor. For example, you may have read articles recently in local newspapers describing a form of gene therapy, in which a virus that is common in the normal population (adenovirus) but is genetically modified to trick cancer cells into accepting materials that may cause malignant cells to die, is described. These and other, almost science-fiction scenarios, are being tried, some of which may one day become the first-line or mainstays of therapy in fighting cancer.

Gene therapy
Treatment that alters a gene. In studies of gene therapy for cancer, researchers are trying to improve the body's natural ability to fight the disease or to make the cancer cells more sensitive to other kinds of therapy by either adding a gene that was lost in the cancer or interfering with a gene that contributes to the growth of the cancer.

On the surgical side, there are novel therapies being tried such as bathing the chest cavity and belly with very hot solutions containing chemotherapy in order to try to kill remaining cells. This experimental procedure is presently under investigation.

By the time you read this book, there will be other molecules and/or treatment strategies that will have entered into clinical trials for mesothelioma at different sites in the United States as well as other countries. You need to ask your doctors specifically about such novel trials, and then decide yourself if you want to participate in those clinical trials after you hear about the possible risks and benefits and, of course, depending upon the various, more standard options that might or might not be available in the treatment of your specific mesothelioma.

67. What is alternative therapy?

Alternative and complementary medicine is the use of remedies or therapies that are not considered part of mainstream medicine. They include a broad range of healing philosophies and approaches such as herbal therapy, acupuncture, meditation, and guided imagery. Although both terms are often used interchangeably, there are slight differences in their meaning. **Alternative therapy** is something that is used in place of or instead of a conventional form of treatment. A complementary therapy is one that is used in addition to rather than in place of a conventional treatment.

Alternative therapy

Practices used instead of standard treatments, which are generally not recognized by the medical community as standard or conventional medical approaches. Alternative medicine includes dietary supplements, megadose vitamins, herbal preparations, special teas, acupuncture, massage therapy, magnet therapy, spiritual healing, and meditation.

68. What should I know about complementary and alternative therapies?

Interest in complementary and alternative therapy has been increasing over the past few years. People diagnosed with many types of diseases, including cancer, are now exploring these options. In the past, there had been very few well-designed studies that looked at the effectiveness and safety of these therapies. What information was available was in the form of anecdotal notes (someone told someone else that the treatment worked).

This seems to be changing now as more research is being done in this area. Most patients who decide to use this type of approach will use a complementary therapy, in other words, one of the alternative therapies used in combination with their conventional treatment. Some people choose to use alternative therapies alone as their treatment, or to use them after all conventional treatment has failed or they perceive them to have failed. Many of these alternative and or complementary therapies are based on some nutritional concept such as a specific diet. The primary goal behind many of these therapies is to try to restore a poorly functioning immune system that is having trouble controlling the growth of the cancer. However, there are conflicting opinions on whether immune system enhancers should be used during active treatment. It is best to talk with your doctor before beginning any type of alternative or complementary therapy. At times, these therapies may interact with the conventional therapy that is prescribed. For example, they may decrease the effectiveness of your treatment or cause more side effects to occur.

69. How do I decide on a treatment plan when faced with multiple options?

Deciding on the best treatment plan for your mesothelioma can be overwhelming, especially when you have been given multiple options. It is in your best interest to take some time to learn about the disease and its treatment. Having a full discussion with your healthcare team about the extent of your disease, the purpose of treatments, any potential side effects, and the expected results is an important part of the process. The best time to obtain a second opinion is during this stage of decision-making, prior to the start of any type of treatment.

Your network of family and friends is invaluable during this time and may be able to assist you in making some of these difficult decisions. Ask both your original doctor and the doctors you see for a second opinion about any clinical trials that may be available for you to participate in. Before you decide on a plan of care, you should understand the differences among the treatments and how they compare to one another in terms of possible side effects, risks, benefits, and impact on your current lifestyle. You may use members of your healthcare team to help you make decisions, but remember, the final choice is yours.

70. How do I know if my treatment is working?

Several different methods are used to determine how well your treatment is working. First, you will be seeing your doctor regularly during this treatment period and will be having frequent physical exams and laboratory tests to look for signs of disease regression, treatment-related side effects, or a possible increase in your disease burden. You will be asked to watch for any unusual or new symptoms and to report any of these to your doctor. If some new symptom develops that involves another site of the body, your doctor will order specific tests (usually radiological studies) to evaluate the area.

Before your treatment started, you had X-rays and CT scans performed to learn the extent and size of your disease. The same types of scans will be repeated at specific intervals to analyze these areas and determine whether your cancer has decreased or increased in size or stayed the same during your treatment. In talking about how well the treatment is working, your doctor will speak in terms of the disease's response to the treatment. **Complete response** means that the cancer appears to be completely gone from the body. **Partial response** means that the tumor has shrunk by at least 50% of its original size. No response or **stable disease** means that the cancer has not really grown or shrunk during the treatment. Lastly, **progressive disease** means that the cancer is growing despite the treatment you have received. By looking at the various test results, the doctor gains valuable information about how effective your treatment has been and can, as a result, discuss with you what, if any, the next step should be.

71. What if my disease has remained stable during treatment?

If your disease has remained stable during your treatment—that is, it has not grown or shrunk—this would imply that the cancer has remained much the same as when you started the therapy. Although the ultimate goal of any treatment plan is to rid the body of all of the cancer or as much of it as is possible, the fact that your cancer has not continued to grow is, especially in the setting of a cancer such as mesothelioma, which can often be quite resistant to any form of therapy, a positive sign. The treatment has at least helped to keep the cancer in check and not allowed it to get any worse. If you are in the middle of your treatment, the doctor will probably have you continue on the same therapy until the planned length of treatment is completed. If you are at the end of your current treatment, a change will likely be advised, as it is most likely that with the discontinuation of any active treatment, the cancer will progress and possibly spread to other sites. It is at this point that you will likely face the issue of considering a clinical trial or

Complete response

The disappearance of all signs of cancer in response to treatment; also called a complete remission. This does not always mean the cancer has been cured.

Partial response

A decrease in the size of a tumor or in the extent of cancer in the body in response to treatment.

Stable disease

Cancer that is neither decreasing nor increasing in extent or severity.

Progressive disease

Cancer that is increasing in scope or severity.

considering a period of rest from any treatment, or the use of an alternative therapy or palliative therapy, as we have previously discussed in this book, depending on your overall health state and frame of mind. Remember that there are no rights or wrongs in the decisions you make at this stage. However, all such decisions should be reached together with family members, caregivers, and other advisers who have helped in your general management up to that time. These decisions also need to be made with a clear understanding of what each option implies and thus, it requires that you be able to think clearly and rationally at such times and not be influenced by depression or the use of too much pain medicine or other medications that might dim your ability to concentrate on the issues at hand. Hopefully, and perhaps above all, your doctors, with whom you have developed a personal trust, can help you make the best decision for your ongoing care. Again, any decision made at this time, whether to do nothing or to move toward a clinical trial, can always be altered at any point should circumstances change.

PART SEVEN

Side Effects of Therapy

What can I do to relieve my pain?

Are there long-term side effects
from treatment?

How should I change my diet following a
mesothelioma diagnosis? Should I
take dietary supplements? Can diet
affect my survival?

What are the benefits of exercise for
mesothelioma patients?

More...

72. Why am I always tired? What can I do for fatigue? Will the fatigue go away after my treatment is over? Could I be depressed?

Fatigue is one of the most common complaints among cancer patients. People will often say that they can't do the things they used to enjoy doing and that this has affected their lifestyle. There is usually no single cause associated with this fatigue; instead a combination of multiple factors leads to this feeling. These include stress related to the illness and its treatment, symptoms of the disease, nutritional changes, psychological factors such as anxiety and fear, and side effects of treatment. In order to understand cancer fatigue, you must first have an understanding of normal fatigue. This type of fatigue occurs in response to strenuous mental or physical activity and has a protective effect that helps prevent injury. The fatigue seen in people with cancer is much more debilitating. It is an overwhelming sense of exhaustion that does not respond easily to rest and persists over time, causing a decreased ability to perform everyday normal activities.

It's important to try to find out what is causing your fatigue so that you know what you're dealing with. Fatigue may be the result of the disease itself or its treatment. Mesothelioma can affect your breathing in a number of ways. You may have had lung surgery that has caused you to lose lung tissue, or your disease may be reducing your breathing capacity. This can lead to fatigue because less oxygen is being taken in and less carbon dioxide is going out of the body. Chemotherapy and radiation therapy can also lead to fatigue. Both of these treatments can affect the bone marrow and its ability to make red blood cells. These cells are responsible for carrying oxygen to the tissues in the body. If you have too few red blood cells (anemia), the body tissues don't get enough oxygen to do their work, and thus you may feel fatigued, weak, short of breath, and/or dizzy. You may require a blood transfusion to increase the number of red blood cells if your levels become too low. It's important to let your doctor know if any of these symptoms occur. Your blood counts will be monitored closely while you are receiving your treatment.

Fatigue can also be the result of stress related to your cancer, trips to the hospital for your treatment, uncontrolled pain, and lack of sleep. Here are some strategies you may want to try to combat this problem:

- Limit the activities you do in a day to those that are most important to you.
- Plan uninterrupted rest periods before and after activities to help conserve your energy.
- Get some light exercise, like taking a walk everyday. This will help to increase your energy level. It can also help maintain your muscle tone.
- Talk with others about your fears and concerns and try to reduce the stresses in your life. You may need to seek professional help from psychiatrists, psychologists, social workers, or others to help in this regard.
- Make sure you are eating as well as you can. A well-balanced diet that consists of several small meals throughout the day is best. Ask to speak to a dietician if you need help in this area.
- Ask for assistance from your healthcare team if you are experiencing pain, or sleep difficulties.

- Don't be afraid to ask for help from your family and friends. They can assist you with things like housework, driving, and shopping.

Fatigue caused by the cancer treatment itself usually declines slowly over a period of a few weeks after its completion. Although cancer-related fatigue is often a challenging problem and frustrating to those experiencing it, there are ways to cope with its effects.

The diagnosis of mesothelioma can be very overwhelming for you and your family members. It is not uncommon to experience depression nor is it a sign of weakness. It is important to recognize the symptoms and to act on them swiftly as you wish to be in the best possible state to make any important decisions and to be an active participant in your medical care. Depression can cause fatigue, lack of appetite, loss of sexual function, lack of desire to socialize with friends and family, and sleep disturbance. These are just a few signals that may lead to the diagnosis of depression. Depression, like your illness, is treatable and should be considered part of overall good medical care. Discuss your symptoms with your medical team and they may recommend counseling or medication to help alleviate some of these symptoms, thus freeing you to focus on more important areas of your life.

73. What can I do about my shortness of breath?

Shortness of breath (SOB) is a common symptom of mesothelioma. A person becomes short of breath when the tissues in his or her body are in need of more oxygen in order to function appropriately. This need for oxygen causes a person to start breathing faster and can lead to a feeling of anxiety. The rapid breathing that may result actually may make the problem worse and starts a cycle that can be hard to break. SOB can be caused by a number of things, including fluid in the space between the lung and chest wall, tumors in the chest that encroach on normal lung tissue, anemia, and muscle weakness. There are also other underlying conditions that may cause this problem, such as chronic obstructive pulmonary disease (COPD), emphysema, heart disease, and depression. Often patients with mesothelioma have one or more of these medical problems that may contribute to their SOB. It is important to determine the actual cause of the SOB because treatment may be available. If it is related to fluid that has accumulated in your chest (pleural effusion), there is a good possibility that this can be drained, often resulting in less SOB. Sometimes an inhaler can help, especially if you have other medical conditions that cause your airways to constrict, such as asthma or COPD. If you already have a pulmonologist, continue to visit with them, as they can be very helpful in managing pulmonary symptoms. There are different forms of anemia, and some may require taking iron pills or a transfusion to correct the condition. Being anemic not only causes SOB, but can result in headaches, anxiety, and fatigue so correcting this situation can certainly contribute positively to your sense of well-being. Lastly, some patients benefit from supplemental oxygen, which today can be delivered from a portable canister, thus allowing you to continue to go outdoors and socialize in restaurants, parks, etc.

The following are some tips to help you manage your SOB:

- Try using relaxation techniques to relax your muscles because when your muscles are tense they use more oxygen. Guided imagery, meditation, and the use of relaxation tapes are further helpful approaches in this regard.
- Take frequent rests when you are walking or performing any physical exercise.
- Sleep on more than one pillow so that your head is raised above your shoulders.
- Let your doctor know if you are experiencing SOB, as he or she may suggest oxygen or medications to help ease your breathing.
- Practice controlled breathing to help you feel as though you are getting enough air. Start with a normal breath and count the seconds it takes you to inhale through your nose. Then exhale normally through pursed lips for twice as long as you inhaled.

74. What can I do to relieve my pain?

Patients with mesothelioma can experience pain and today we have many new types of drugs that can significantly reduce the amount of pain that you may experience. Pain can be described as acute, meaning that it comes on suddenly and resolves in a short period of time. Chronic pain refers to pain that can persist for months and even years and requires good management as adjustments in the doses and types of medications might be necessary. If your pain is related to your surgical procedure, you will continue to take your pain medication as prescribed until it has resolved or becomes more tolerable. If you experience a new onset of pain, or pain in a new area, you will need to schedule an appointment with your physician to determine the source of your pain and thus find a means of resolving it. We have pain medications that are given orally, transdermally (delivered by a patch that you place on your skin), rectally, or intravenously, or by injections administered into the skin, spinal fluid, or nerves. These are just a few examples of methods that we can use to attack your pain. If pain is localized to a specific area that can be irradiated, you might be referred to a radiation oncologist to direct therapy to the precise location of your pain. This can be very beneficial in some situations. Patients may experience nerve-related pain (neuropathic pain), which can be described as shooting or burning pain and can be the result of nerve injury from your cancer, chemotherapy, surgery, or radiation therapy (neuropathic pain). We now have special classes of drugs that have been found to be more effective in controlling this type of pain than traditional pain medication. Often patients may be prescribed a combination of pain medications, as the pain may be multifactorial. We usually suggest that you make a specific appointment to meet with your medical team specifically to focus on your pain management. This will ensure that you will have the full attention of your medical team in helping to resolve this pressing problem. Keep a pain diary at home listing the type of pain, location, severity, and duration of pain using a recognized pain scale. Also record which drugs, if any, help and for how long. This information will help to guide the doctor in prescribing medications using a more personalized approach. Taking prescribed pain medications can help you to take back control of your life and engage in more pleasurable activities. When your pain is not well managed, you can become depressed, experience fatigue, have personality changes (become grumpy or anxious), and have trouble maintaining your daily activity schedule, thus causing you to withdraw from some of the activities that you may have enjoyed in the past. Some patients are under the impression that they have to worry about addiction or that people will think less of them when they are taking pain medications, but this is based on outdated social norms. We refer to pain as the fifth vital sign and your medical team has been educated on the need to assess pain and to intervene when appropriate. The experience of pain can change throughout the illness and you will most likely require periodic adjustments in your pain medication to keep it under control. At times, you may even be able to stop taking, or significantly reduce, the dose of pain medications if your pain is resolved by one or all of the treatments you receive in the management of your mesothelioma.

You can play an important role in controlling your pain by expressing your feelings and describing the pain to your healthcare team. Remember that treating pain right away is more effective than waiting until it becomes more severe. Also remember that there is no need for you to experience any pain or pain for any length of time. A *very* important part of the management of cancer is to prevent or treat pain and your medical team should be cognizant of this. Many hospitals have pain teams or clinics that specialize in the treatment of pain and your doctor may send you to see these professionals. Sometimes pain can't be controlled with medications, and other treatments such as nerve blocks to block pain due to nerve compression, surgery, or radiation used to shrink the tumor can be used. The main goal of any pain regimen is to control pain with the maximum amount of relief and minimal side effects. Your doctor will work with you to find the most effective treatment for your individual pain needs. The major complications of most pain medications, since they are usually some form of narcotic agent, can be drowsiness to the point of confusion, constipation, or nausea. All of these issues can be avoided or resolved. Becoming addicted to pain medications is *not* an issue in patients with cancer, as you will easily be able to stop these medications once the actual cause of your pain is resolved.

75. What can I do to prevent or relieve constipation?

Constipation is a common side effect that occurs in people who are taking narcotic pain medications or who are receiving chemotherapy treatment for their cancer. Contributing to the problem is the fact that you may be less active and may not eating as well as you normally would. It is important to drink plenty of fluids and stick to high-fiber foods such as fruits and vegetables, nuts, and whole-wheat breads and cereals. Try to avoid foods that can cause constipation, such as cheese. Don't forget about those old-time remedies, such as prunes or prune juice and bran. If possible, exercise by simply getting outside and taking a walk. You may need to take stool softeners and/or laxatives on a daily basis, especially if you are taking narcotic pain medications. Be sure to take these as recommended and not just when you feel you need them. In some cases, if these remedies are not effective, you may require an enema or suppository. Let your doctor know if you haven't had a bowel movement in three or more days, and check with him or her before taking any of these remedies.

SIDE EFFECTS OF THERAPY

76. Am I at risk for a blood clot? What is a pulmonary embolism?

People diagnosed with cancers such as mesothelioma may be more prone to developing blood clots. This is because they can have more platelets (cells that cause the blood to clot) in their bloodstream than normal. Also, they may be more debilitated and may not be getting up and moving around enough. Often, blood clots form in the legs and cause the legs and feet to become red, swollen, and/or tender. Blood clots can be very serious since once they occur, they have the ability to move through the bloodstream to other organs, such as the lungs, heart, or rarely the brain, depending on where the clot is located. If a clot breaks off from a site in the legs, it may travel to the lung, causing a pulmonary embolism. This is a blockage of the lung artery or one of its branches. A pulmonary embolism can be fatal so it is very important to identify and treat blood clots in the extremities as soon as possible. If not fatal, a pulmonary embolism usually causes sudden chest pain, which is usually described as worse on breathing deeply, and/or the sudden onset of SOB, often to the point where you become unable to move around. Blood clots can be treated with medications that cause the blood to become thin (anticoagulated), and therefore reducing the chance of a clot developing or preventing an established clot from embolizing (breaking off and travelling to the lung). Heparin, or one if its newer derivatives, is the injectable drug that is used initially, followed by the use of oral coumadin. While on coumadin, you will require frequent blood tests to make sure you are receiving the right amount of the drug. Because of this risk of blood clots, make sure to report any symptoms of swelling in the legs and feet or any sudden onset of SOB or chest pain to your doctor immediately.

77. Will I have terrible nausea and vomiting during my chemotherapy treatment?

For many years, chemotherapy has been automatically associated with nausea and vomiting. Although these side effects are common, not all chemotherapy drugs cause nausea and vomiting and not every person will experience these symptoms to the same extent. It is true that these drugs are very powerful and many of them can cause nausea, episodes of vomiting, or both. However, there are a number of new medications on the market today that control nausea and vomiting much more effectively than their older counterparts did. Preventing nausea and vomiting is much easier than trying to get it under control once it happens. Therefore, before you even start your chemotherapy treatment, you will be given antinausea medications to help prevent you from getting sick. Chemotherapy can affect the stomach, the vomiting control center in the brain, or both. A wide variety of drugs is available to control or lessen these effects. Not all drugs work the same for all people, and it may be necessary to change the drug you use or combine more than one antinausea drug to provide the best and most complete relief. Some people experience slight nausea most of the time, while others become severely nauseated for only a limited time period after the chemotherapy administration. Symptoms may start soon after treatment or 8–12 hours later and may last only a few hours or up to 24 hours after the therapy is given. Some people may even start to feel sick before their treatment starts; this is known as **anticipatory nausea and vomiting (ANV)**, which is more usually psychological or due to the expectation that you will become nauseated and vomit. It is important to let your doctor or nurses know if you are experiencing severe nausea or have vomited for

Anticipatory nausea and vomiting (ANV)

ANV is nausea and/or vomiting that occur prior to the beginning of a new cycle of chemotherapy in response to conditioned stimuli such as the smells, sights, and sounds of the treatment room. ANV is a classically conditioned response that typically occurs after 3 or 4 prior chemotherapy treatments, following which the person experienced acute or delayed nausea and vomiting.

more than a day. If you are unable to keep liquids down, you may become dehydrated and need to have fluids given to you intravenously. Severe dehydration may even require you to be hospitalized. Here are some suggestions for ways to limit your symptoms:

- Try eating small, frequent meals throughout the day so your stomach doesn't feel too full.
- Eat your meals slowly and drink fluids at least an hour before or after your meals instead of with them.
- Avoid strong odors such as perfume or cooking smells.
- Wear clothing that is loose and doesn't bind.
- Distract yourself by using relaxation techniques or by watching television or listening to music while you eat as well as during your periods of rest.
- Eat foods cold or at room temperature and avoid fried, sweet, or fatty foods or those that are strong tasting.
- If you are nauseated, try eating mild foods, such as crackers or toast.

Recent studies have reported the benefit of ginger in controlling nausea. You may want to consider adding it to your antinausea regimen. Talk with your healthcare provider and work with him or her to find the treatment that is best for you.

78. Will I lose my hair during chemotherapy or radiation?

Hair loss is another common side effect of cancer treatment and can be one of the most psychologically traumatic. Although it's not harmful to the body, it is a constant visual reminder of the effects of cancer and its treatment and can significantly alter the way you look and fell about yourself. Your doctor can tell you whether the chemotherapy drugs you will receive are likely to cause hair loss. Alopecia (hair loss) occurs because chemotherapy kills hair follicles, and thus hair falls out more quickly than normal. If hair loss does occur, certain areas such as the head or the entire body may be affected, including the eyelashes and eyebrows. The hair can become thinner or it can be lost completely. Hair loss will usually begin anywhere from one week to several weeks after treatment and may occur gradually or in clumps.

Hair loss associated with chemotherapy is usually temporary. Your hair will start to grow back after your treatments are over, but it may take four to six months following the completion of your treatment for it to do so. Sometimes it may even start to grow back while you are still receiving your chemotherapy. The new hair may be a different texture, color, or thickness when it grows back, but these changes are not usually permanent.

Radiation therapy can also cause hair thinning or loss of hair, but it does not occur over the entire body. Only the area that is directly under the radiation beam will be affected. Therefore, if you are receiving radiation to your chest, the hair loss will occur on your chest area only. The hair on your head will be affected only if you are receiving radiation to your head or scalp. Hair may start to fall out two to three weeks after the radiation starts. Usually it will start to grow back after radiation treatments are completed, but if the dose of radiation you received was high, the hair loss may be partially or completely permanent.

Before treatment begins, you may want to look into buying a wig or hairpiece. This is often covered by insurance so be sure to ask your physician for a prescription for a hair prosthesis. This is the best time to see a professional hairdresser or wig consultant because he or she will be able to match the color and style of the wig or hair piece to your real hair. The American Cancer Society has wigs that they loan to people, so if this interests you, give them a call. It might be helpful to have your hair cut shorter to make hair loss easier to manage if it should happen. Some people try wearing bandanas, scarves, or hats. These are all ways to help you feel normal during your cancer treatment. Do what feels most comfortable for you. During your chemotherapy, try to use mild shampoos, soft hairbrushes, and low heat when using a hair dryer, and avoid the use of hair dye. Losing your hair can be difficult and can cause you to feel angry or depressed. Talking about your feelings with those you trust may help.

79. Is my cough something I should worry about?

A cough is one of the symptoms that can occur with mesothelioma, and it can result from fluid pressing on the lung or from the tumor mass irritating the pleura. A change in the pattern of an existing cough may be an important warning sign and should be followed up on. During the course of your illness, the underlying reason for your cough may change. This is why it is necessary to let your doctor know about any differences in an underlying cough as soon as they happen. In order to treat your cough as effectively as possible, it is important to identify the cause.

As we noted previously, your cough may be caused by fluid that is around your lung in the pleural space. If your doctor performs a procedure to remove this fluid, your cough may improve or disappear. However, if your cough returns or becomes worse, this may be one of the first signs that the fluid has come back and/or cancer recurred or progressed. Your doctor may order a chest X-ray to evaluate the situation and may perform another procedure to try to get rid of the fluid. When no specific, treatable cause for the cough is found, the doctor may prescribe a cough suppressant.

80. What can I do if I have lost my appetite?

Mesothelioma and its treatment can cause a loss of normal appetite (**anorexia**). There are a number of specific reasons why you may lose your appetite. These include tumor growth, depression, difficulty swallowing, pain, nausea, and changes in taste and smell. Chemotherapy can cause the normal cells that line your mouth, stomach, and intestines to be altered or destroyed. This may, in turn, cause the food and fluids that you take in to taste different. They may take on a metallic or bitter taste, or may seem very sweet. You may also lose your desire to eat but this is usually temporary and improves over a period of two to six weeks after your chemotherapy has been completed.

Anorexia

An abnormal loss of the appetite for food. Anorexia can be caused by cancer, AIDS, a mental disorder (such as anorexia nervosa), or other diseases.

It is very important for you to eat as much as you can in order to maintain your weight. Those who eat well seem to be able to cope better and fight off infection easier. If you find something that tastes good and you can eat it without difficulty, then do so. Eat anything you want and as much as you want. A list of suggestions to help you manage your loss of appetite follows this paragraph. Prior to your diagnosis of cancer, you may have been placed on a cholesterol-lowering diet. In times of serious illness or with certain medications, many previous food restrictions are no longer appropriate. It makes sense to schedule an appointment with your primary care doctor or oncologist to determine what medications continue to be necessary and what dietary modifications, if any, would now be recommended. Oatmeal, which has become a popular breakfast choice, adds few calories, but much bulk and can thus create a sense of fullness, which may interfere with your ability to take in extra needed calories.

- Snack frequently throughout the day, and eat whenever you feel like you can.
- Eat high-calorie and high-protein foods and snacks, such as nuts, eggs, peanut butter, and milkshakes. Try adding protein powders to drinks.
- Add butter or margarine, creams, and gravies to your meals to boost calories.
- Let other people fix your meals so you are able to conserve energy and stay away from cooking odors.
- Do some light exercise, like walking, about an hour before you eat to stimulate your appetite.
- Drink plenty of fluids but try to drink them between meals instead of with them because they can contribute to your feelings of fullness.
- If your food tastes metallic, use plastic utensils instead of metal.
- Eat with friends or family whenever possible, as socializing helps to increase appetite. When you are eating alone, watch TV or have the radio on to distract you.

- Vary your mealtime routine and try new foods and recipes.
- Use food supplements like Ensure if you are able to. They are high in calories and nutrients.

Anorexia can lead to a very serious problem for people with cancer called **cachexia**, which is a condition that causes a breakdown in muscle mass in those with chronic illness. Weight loss is a symptom of cancer and a side effect of treatment, but if left unchecked, it can lead to cachexia. Your doctor may consider starting you on medications, like Megace, anabolic steroids, or other appetite stimulants, to help increase your appetite if you appear to be losing too much weight and becoming cachexic. Be sure to discuss any appetite problems with your doctor, and notify him or her if you are losing weight.

Cachexia

Loss of body weight and muscle mass, and weakness that may occur in patients with cancer, AIDS, or other chronic diseases. Cachexia is a common manifestation of late-stage mesothelioma.

81. Are there long-term side effects from treatment?

Most side effects that are experienced as a result of surgery resolve in a few days to a few weeks after the operation. Pain, however, is one side effect that may last for longer periods of time. Pain at the incision site is an expected outcome of chest surgery, but some people complain of lasting pain that is sometimes harder to eliminate. You will be provided with effective pain medication that you will continue to take at home when you are discharged. Your doctor will work with you to find the most effective medications to help relieve any discomfort that you may have. It is often helpful to involve a pain specialist to help you in managing your pain, especially in the situation in which the pain becomes a more chronic feature of your existence. Having your pain effectively controlled greatly contributes to your quality of life and your ability to fight this disease.

Chemotherapy and radiation work to destroy cancer cells but also damage normal cells, especially those that divide more rapidly, at the same time. Fortunately, normal cells recover quickly and side effects gradually disappear after treatment ends. The length of time it takes to feel better and regain your energy may vary in different people. Many times, side effects go away very quickly but certain ones may take months or years to recede completely. It is important to discuss any side effects you may be having with your medical team. Often patients are reluctant to bring them up for fear of having their chemotherapy discontinued. In most cases, we can prescribe medications to diminish these side effects and sometimes we will change your current treatment if it is thought that the risks of a particular therapy outweigh the potential benefits. Remember this is a team effort and an open and honest relationship is important for your safety and well-being. Other times, the treatment may cause side effects that result in permanent damage and can last a lifetime. Sometimes chemotherapy can cause permanent damage to the lungs, kidneys, or heart, depending on the type of chemotherapy you receive and your body's response to it. A specific side effect of chemotherapy, peripheral neuropathy, may cause difficulty with balance or gait and can also make it difficult to pick up and manipulate objects. If you develop a peripheral neuropathy, the symptoms may improve after the completion of chemotherapy, but they might not totally go away.

It is important to keep in mind that many people don't experience any long-term problems. The unwanted effects of treatment may not be pleasant, but they must be compared to the benefits of treatment and its ability to destroy the cancer. Talk with your doctor or nurse if you have any questions about side effects or the way you are feeling after treatment.

82. How should I change my diet following a mesothelioma diagnosis? Should I take dietary supplements? Can diet affect my survival?

Eating well, although it can be challenging at times, enables you to cope better with the disease and its treatment. It is important that you drink a lot of fluids and eat as much as you can so that you are able to maintain your weight and strength. This means that you should pick a variety of foods that contain protein, calories, vitamins, and minerals to keep your body functioning properly. Protein-enriched foods help build and repair body tissues that are injured. If your calorie intake is too low, the body uses protein for energy first, and there may not be enough left to repair the tissues.

Cancer is known to affect a person's metabolism, even though the mechanism for this is not clear. Some nutrition experts say that during treatment a person may require up to 50% more protein and 20% more calories than normal. It has been shown that patients who are able to eat and drink well are better able to handle the side effects of treatment and can fight off infection more easily by strengthening the immune system. Also, it can make a big difference in a person's outlook and quality of life.

Nutritional supplements may help fill the gap in nutrients that are missing from your diet. This gap may be due to a lack of appetite or depletion of key nutrients because of stress or certain medications you are on. Some people may benefit from taking vitamin and mineral supplements, but before doing so, you should check with your doctor. High doses of certain vitamins and minerals can be **toxic** or can react adversely with treatment medications. Ask to speak to a dietician if you have specific nutritional questions or need assistance with your diet.

Toxic

Having to do with poison or something harmful to the body. Toxic substances usually cause unwanted side effects.

83. What are the benefits of exercise for mesothelioma patients?

Exercise is an important consideration for all people, whether they are currently healthy and disease-free or are diagnosed with cancer and undergoing treatment. You may already have a regular exercise routine that you follow, and if you have surgery, your doctors should encourage you to get back into that or some other exercise routine. If you are able to continue with your previous routine, then do so; however, you may find it necessary to adjust it somewhat. Keep in mind that any type of light exercise is useful and may help to decrease your feelings of fatigue and stimulate your appetite. Walking is an exercise that is usually well tolerated, and you should walk as much as possible. One way you can give your arms some exercise is by lifting light weights. If the muscles in your chest and arms are sore, you can also use exercises such as slow stretching or "walking" your fingers up a wall to relieve this. It is important to talk with your doctor before starting on any exercise program. If you are feeling weak and have lost muscle strength, you might request a prescription for physical therapy to strengthen and tone your body. They can work with you to develop a program of exercise tailored to your medical status.

84. What about returning to work?

Work is an important part of life for many people and can provide a sense of purpose and financial security. Also, many psychological and social needs are met at the workplace.

Some people who are diagnosed with mesothelioma are able to return to work at some point, either during or after treatment. Your doctor may place restrictions on the activities or job duties that you can perform based on limitations you may have. When returning to work, you may also be faced with issues such as how to talk about your disease and its treatment with coworkers and how to deal with their reactions. It might be helpful for you to plan ahead and work through some of these concerns beforehand. The American with Disabilities Act protects workers, including those diagnosed with cancer. You may want to check with your legal advisor prior to returning to the workplace. Discuss your individual needs and work situation with your doctor. He or she will let you know if and when you can return to work and will help in any way possible.

85. What about follow-up care? How often should I be seen?

All patients with mesothelioma who receive treatment should be monitored very closely during and after treatment, whether they participate in a clinical trial or not. If you are on a specific clinical trial, the follow-up schedule will be clearly defined in the protocol and will be explained to you before you start the trial. During treatment with chemotherapy, most patients will have weekly blood levels drawn and will be seen by the doctor every two to three weeks. You will receive a physical examination and blood work when you come to see the doctor and will be asked to report any new symptoms you may be having.

A CT scan will usually be performed after two cycles of chemotherapy to see how the cancer is responding to the treatment. If your cancer appears to be getting worse, the doctor will stop the chemotherapy that you are receiving and develop a new plan. If you complete all the treatment you were to receive, the doctor will perform another CT scan and will again evaluate the tumor's response to the treatment. When your therapy has been completed, you will still be monitored with CT scans at regular intervals, along with follow-up visits with your doctor.

In between visits, you need to notify your doctor of any new problems you may be experiencing as soon as they develop. Depending on the symptom you are having, your doctor may order a CT scan earlier than you normally would have one, to evaluate for any possible cancer recurrence or growth. If your cancer returns or becomes worse, you may have to receive more treatment. Your doctor will discuss your options with you at that time.

There is a large effort underway to study survivorship in cancer patients. Once your therapy has been completed, you may consider seeing a specialist in survivorship issues. These specialty clinics are just getting started in many of the university-based hospitals.

86. Should I get a flu shot or pneumonia vaccine?

Yearly flu shots are recommended for anyone who is 50 years of age or older or has a chronic illness and whose immune system may be compromised. People with a diagnosis of cancer fall into this category and are encouraged to ask their doctor for a flu shot every year. If you have never received the pneumonia vaccine in the past, it is a good idea to receive this vaccine as well. If you have received the pneumonia vaccine before, you will be asked how long ago you received it. If it has been five years or more, you should be vaccinated again. It is currently recommended that a person receive only two lifetime doses of the vaccine, so if you have had it twice already, you do not need to repeat it.

PART EIGHT

Recurrence of the Disease

What happens if my disease recurs?

Where is my disease likely to recur?

How is recurrence treated?

More...

87. *What happens if my disease recurs?*

No one can predict when your disease may recur, but it is important for patients and those involved with your care to be alert for the signs of recurrence and to keep abreast of the latest developments in the treatment of mesothelioma. There are some symptoms that are highly suspicious for a recurrence of disease. Night sweats are often one of the first symptoms experienced by mesothelioma patients. In many patients, night sweats will disappear following surgery or when chemotherapy has been effective. If you have a return of night sweats, increasing shortness of breath, pain, abdominal girth, weight loss, or any unexplained change in your feeling of wellness, you should contact your healthcare team. I would advise that you not wait for your regularly scheduled follow-up visit, but call and ascertain if you should be evaluated at an earlier date.

When cancer recurs, it becomes active again in the body after a period of inactivity or dormancy. This can happen quickly over weeks or months, or it can take longer and occur years later. **Recurrent cancers** begin with abnormal cells that start to grow and multiply quickly, much like the original cancer. These recurrent tumors start from cells that originated from the first cancer. These cells were either left behind after treatment was completed, either because they were too small to see or because they broke away from the primary tumor and traveled through the lymphatic system or bloodstream to other parts of the body.

Recurrent cancers are classified by location because not only do they differ in their ability to recur, but they also differ in the place where they are likely to recur.

Recurrent cancer
Cancer that has returned after a period of time during which the cancer could not be detected. The cancer can come back to the same site as the original (primary) tumor or to another place in the body.

In pleural mesothelioma, if your disease were to recur in the abdomen, we would still classify your disease as pleural mesothelioma noting that it has metastasized to the abdomen. If the cancer has returned to the same area of the body that it started in, it is called a **local recurrence**. It also means that it is isolated to that area and has not spread to other tissues. A cancer, that involves new growth in nearby lymph nodes or tissues near the original site of the cancer, is called a **regional recurrence**. Lastly, if the cancer is now found in other organs or tissues that are at some distance from the original site, it is called a **metastatic recurrence**. The treatment you receive now will depend on many factors, including where the disease has recurred, what treatments are available, and your overall health status.

88. Where is my disease likely to recur?

Mesothelioma is a disease that likes to come back to the same area that it originated in. Therefore, if it was first diagnosed in your chest cavity, that is where it will most likely return. The other problem with the disease is that it likes to grow in old wound sites. This process is known as **malignant seeding** and is a common complication of procedures performed on patients with mesothelioma. The areas that your doctor needs to monitor for any signs of possible recurrence include thoracentesis tracts, biopsy tracts, chest-tube sites, and surgical incisions. This is why your doctor will ask to feel and look at these sites during your physical exams. Also, be sure to alert your doctor to any new or abnormal lumps or bumps that you notice in these areas. Spread to distant metastatic sites can occur, but this usually happens late in the course of the disease.

Local recurrence

Reappearance of the previously treated cancer at its original site; with mesothelioma, a local recurrence occurs in the pleura most frequently after surgery for the tumor.

Regional recurrence

Return of the cancer in a location close to the original cancer.

Metastatic recurrence

Return of the cancer at a site away from the original site.

Malignant seeding

Growth of a tumor at a site that may be outside its original domain because of contamination of a new site with malignant cells after a biopsy or from cells in a malignant effusion.

After treatment in the chest, the disease can start to grow in the belly. Difficulty in closing skirts or pants at the waist, loss of appetite, and a feeling of fullness can be the harbinger that fluid is building up in the abdomen and that the disease has spread there.

It is important that you follow up with your doctor and are monitored on a regular basis. You should be having CT scans performed at regular intervals after your treatment is completed in order to evaluate your progress and to check for any possible local or more distant recurrence.

89. How is recurrence treated?

If your disease recurs, your doctor will discuss what treatments are now available for you. The treatment options will depend on the size and location of your cancer, what treatments you have already received, and your overall health status. The types of treatments that are recommended to you may include surgery, chemotherapy, or radiation therapy. You should discuss the options thoroughly with your doctor, including what the goals of treatment are and what the possible effects may be.

If your initial chemotherapy regimen was successful and the recurrence occurs some time after the cessation of any therapy, oftentimes you may be re-treated with the same regimen if you are able to tolerate the same drugs. If you recur in a short period of time after completing your previous treatment course, alternative drugs or strategies will likely be discussed.

Surgery is usually reserved for those people who have recurrences at previous incision sites. It might be possible for your surgeon to remove these local recurrences as long as there is no evidence of spread to any other areas. Sometimes surgery is followed by radiation therapy to that area to try to kill cells that may have been left behind. If you have had a PD or EPP and your chest remains stable, you may be referred to a peritoneal surgeon to evaluate the role of surgery and chemotherapy if the disease recurs in the abdomen. This should only be considered under the guidance of a mesothelioma expert, as there are many factors that need to be taken into consideration prior to exposing a patient to the risks associated with possible extensive abdominal surgery. It is always a fine balance between the benefits and risks of any procedure, and the goal in the setting of recurrent disease, just as with your primary therapy, is to provide you with the best quality of life for the longest time possible.

Ask your doctor or consult with the medical liaison at the Meso Foundation to tell you about any clinical trials that are available, as new studies may have opened since your original diagnosis. You may have to prepare yourself to travel, as clinical trials vary from center to center. It is not uncommon to see more than one specialist at this time, as you might want to line up a number of options to treat this and potentially future recurrences. Many people who have faced these decisions a second time have said that knowledge and understanding were again key factors in assisting them through the decision-making process. Find out all you can about your cancer and the options you have so you can make informed decisions and meet this challenge head-on again.

RECURRENCE OF THE DISEASE

PART NINE

Sarah's and Sarah Ann's Insights for Care Providers

How do I discuss mesothelioma with children?

How do I maintain a normal life when a family member has mesothelioma?

How do I balance all of the responsibilities?

More...

90. *How do I discuss mesothelioma with children?*

Sarah (mother) says…

Phil and I had several conversations of what was the best way to tell Sarah Ann of his diagnosis of mesothelioma. We knew that there was a very strong possibility that she would lose her father in a few months. At this time we had no idea that Phil would survive 10 years after his diagnosis of mesothelioma! It was a very difficult time for Phil and me to deal with and to have to sit down with a child was heart-wrenching. As much as we were hurting, it was harder looking at Sarah Ann and telling her about this terrible cancer, but we had a very strong family bond and felt that the best way to survive this would be doing it in unity and together, we could help each other to get through this.

Sarah Ann (daughter) adds…

I remember the first time we spoke about my dad's diagnosis. I was 10 years old and my parents sat me down at our dining room table. They told me they had something important to tell me. They wanted me to know that we were a family, and I could always go to them to talk or to ask questions. They asked me if I understood that dad had been sick, and then they went on to tell me that they had just found out how sick he was and what was wrong with him. They told me dad had cancer. At the time I didn't fully understand what cancer was, and the only reference I could make to cancer was that my principal had just passed away from it a couple of years prior. I can remember sitting there watching my mom cry and holding back tears myself because I wanted to stay strong in front of my dad. We decided that night that we were going through the process as a family and we were all in it together. Being open and honest with each other helped me to understand what my dad was going through and the severity of it all. I was able to confide in and grieve with my family, which in the end, I believe brought us closer and helped create the bond we had and that my mom and I still have today.

Every child is different and I would suggest that you check with your family doctor or school counselor to know what would be appropriate for your child.

I was a very curious child and I wanted to know everything. I wanted to be able to understand what was going on at all times and be able to hold a conversation with any adult. I understood at the time my parents were only going to tell me so much because I was very young, but they did tell me what I asked about and the important things I needed to know. As I got older they were able to confide in me more. My parents and I had an understanding from the beginning. If the information they were telling me upset me too much or was too much for me to handle, I just had to let them know and they could cut back. I think it is very important to be open with your children. They are going to worry no matter what you do to shield them and I know that the more information I knew, the more comfort I was able to have in the situation as a whole. Honesty is the best policy and keeping your child informed will help them to feel a part of the process and let them have some sense of control. They don't need to know every detail but the crucial parts are very important to share.

91. Where do I turn for support in dealing with my own stress and anxiety?

Sarah says…

The first people to turn to, naturally, will be your family, but don't sell your caregivers short on their ability to try to help you cope. Sometimes the doctor is not available, but the nurse practitioners are there for you to hear your own problems and help you to work through them. Your local physician, who has known the family for a long time, is also a great source for psychological support, and he may recommend somebody to see who is a family therapist or psychologist. If there is a need for antianxiety medications in order to deal with the situation, deal with one physician who can prescribe these mediations for you and monitor your reaction.

92. What about those inevitable middle-of-the-night situations when my loved one is in pain or has other medical complications?

Sarah says...

It is important to ask your doctor about coverage when he is away and also what to do in the case of an emergency. Oftentimes our specialists were out of town, and in an emergency, you will be taken to the nearest hospital. Take your card that lists your providers as well as your medication list. The physician on call, with this information, can contact your medical team and begin treatment.

93. How do I maintain a normal life when a family member has mesothelioma?

Sarah says...

Normal takes on a whole new meaning after a cancer diagnosis. You have to learn to live life a little differently to survive it. Before cancer, we spent our time doing regular everyday routines, like going to work, school, ball games, grocery shopping, and many other petty things, but once cancer strikes, things change a bit. You now find yourself worrying about the next CT scan results or if the chemotherapy is working.

You always have cancer hanging over your head. You have to find ways to occupy your time and your mind so that it doesn't consume your every thought or you won't survive it— or at least survive it in one piece. I found that attending a support group for caregivers was helpful. Talking with other people experiencing the same problems as myself helped me to remember I was not the only one dealing with cancer.

A lifesaver for me was during Phil's surgery. He met another patient who had mesothelioma and had his surgery 1 day before Phil. I met his wife and we have stayed in touch with each other for the whole 10 years. She has been there for me and truly can say she understands how I feel and what I am going through. I also have close family members that I can talk to and that help Sarah Ann and myself through the difficult times.

Sarah Ann adds...

I think God blessed me with not being athletic because it saved a lot of time that parents normally would be devoting to their kids and allowed my parents to focus on my dad's health. Life will never be completely normal when a loved one has mesothelioma. I do suggest an extensive collection of DVDs and a lot of family time on the couch watching movies and playing games. My dad and I became movie buffs and our favorite ones to watch were the murder mysteries. We spent countless hours watching movies because it was one thing that we were both capable of doing and a great way for us to bond. It's the simple things that I took for granted, like his recipe for his pepperoni roll or this cheese dip during football season. Stop worrying about having a normal life because, in reality, how many people actually have a normal life and what exactly is a normal life? Focus on time and make the best of it. Spend as much time as you can with your loved one. Find a way to have fun so you don't always have to dwell on cancer. That is the best way to maintain some kind of normalcy in a crazy situation. Stop dwelling on cancer and enjoy what you have.

94. How do I balance all of the responsibilities?

Often times caregivers find themselves overwhelmed with all of the responsibilities and demands of caring for a loved one. This disease did not only happen to your loved one but to you as well. Seek professional help as this is a new experience and you may need help managing depression and/or anxiety. It is not selfish to care for yourself. You will be a better caregiver, in better shape, to meet the demands of this new role and still find ways to find satisfaction and happiness in your life. For social support, the Meso Foundation has regularly scheduled teleconferences that connect you with other caregivers who understand what you are going through and can share important tips that they learned during this journey.

Sarah adds…

It is not possible to do everything yourself, especially when you are dealing with mesothelioma. Even on a good day things can be overwhelming. It is helpful to recognize the fact that you need help from time-to-time, and it is okay to ask for it. There were times when Phil was in the hospital that I was there all day and into the evening. I needed someone to pick Sarah Ann up from school and we also had a pet that needed to be fed and taken care of. Our family was more than ready to help with anything we needed. By allowing them to help, it took that stress off my shoulders and allowed me to be with Phil and take care of him. It also helped our family members to feel they could help us.

Sarah Ann adds…

One life lesson my dad instilled in me, and that I try very hard to abide by, is to try and uphold your responsibilities and never let the important things wait. Learning to balance responsibilities became a life style. I grew up with dad being sick and dealing with it became my routine. There wasn't a secret plan that I lived by; it was my life and it became normal to me. As I got older and dad's health started to deteriorate (for example, in my college years), my dad trumped all. If dad was sick and in the hospital, I was there! My family was the most important thing. There would always be time to make up a class, but I knew I wasn't able to make up the days I spent with my dad.

Sarah adds…

Don't even begin to think of doing it all yourself. Allow supportive family and friends to assist. If they offer, say, "Yes, please!" And when in need, ask for assistance.

I quickly quit apologizing for a less-than pristine house and for not having coffee or food to serve when visitors came. Those who did visit were not there for inspections or sustenance of any kind! Family and friends recognize that you have more than enough to keep you busy.

Recently I read in a local newspaper about a wonderful foundation called Cleaning for a Reason, which is available to many cancer patients throughout the country. They provide cleaning assistance—as they describe it, "one less thing to worry about." For more information, go to their Web site at http://cleaningforareason.org. If your community is not on their list, it might be possible to change that with a few phone calls! This foundation also accepts contributions.

95. What else can I do to make my loved one comfortable?

Sarah says...

It became difficult for Phil to pull clothes over his head, so we found it to be easier on him to wear button-up shirts and zipper jackets. That eliminated the need to exert the extra energy of pulling something over his head. It can also be helpful to get a long-handled shoehorn to help with putting shoes on and a long-handled brush to help with showers. There were certain things he preferred to take with him if he was admitted to the hospital so we kept a bag packed at home ready to go. We took things like house shoes, chapstick, clippers, etc.

Sarah Ann adds...

My dad became sick when I was young so at that time, there wasn't a lot for me to do to help out. I did my best to help my mom around the house and tried to stay out of trouble and just hang out with my dad as much as possible. As I got older, I was able to contribute more. I was always very open with my dad about my life and it was a great way for us to bond. Letting my dad in my life gave him a sense of ease. He was more comfortable with his illness and knowing that his health was deteriorating because he knew who I was and what I wanted in life and that I was on the right track to succeeding in my dreams. The only thing my dad ever wanted for me was to be happy and achieve what I wanted out of life (and not to make some of the same mistakes he made). It gave him a lot of comfort to know all of those goals were being met.

Sometimes comfort doesn't come in materialistic things; it comes with joy and peace of mind and that is how I feel I contributed as a young child and as a young adult.

96. How can family and friends help without intruding?

Sarah Ann says...

I have always been more of an independent person. I never really shared a lot with my family or friends about how my dad's illness affected me and to be sitting here answering some of these questions is out of character for me. I didn't really want my family and friends to talk about my dad's illness with me and when my dad was in the hospital, I handled it best if I was left alone and able to process everything that was happening on my own. I know that each person is different and each person's needs vary; this is just what worked for me. I didn't really want to converse with anyone; I just wanted to think. I love my family and friends very much and they were all there for me if and when I needed them. They were always there for my dad and I am very thankful for that. I know for me, the best way my family and friends could help was with a simple hug and talking to me about other things like school or my boyfriend.

Sarah adds...

Visiting a person that is terminally ill can be a little difficult. There are times when a person might feel good and would enjoy a visit because you can feel cut off from people at times. There are other days when they are not feeling well and an unexpected visit can be difficult because you don't want to hurt anyone's feelings. It is a good idea to call ahead, and, while visiting, if you notice the person is getting tired or sleepy, just cut your visit short. Cards, a text message, or even a voice message can be uplifting to not only the person who is sick, but to the caregiver and other family members.

Ask what might help. Let the patient and his or her care provider know that you want them to be direct with you about what's helpful and what isn't. Call ahead before visiting at home or at the hospital. Keep visits brief and upbeat. When you sense that your loved one is tiring or needing to tend to personal care, depart.

Avoid emotional issues or difficult conversations that will add to the patient's stress and anxiety. If a sensitive conversation needs to occur, talk with the care provider first to determine when and how best to approach it.

97. What specific things can family and friends do to assist?

Sarah says...

Preparing a dinner. There were times we spent most of the day having a chemotherapy treatment or having tests and it was nice to come home and not have to spend hours preparing dinner.

Visiting with the patient's family. I had a good friend and family members that would come and sit with me in the waiting room to keep me company in between the intensive care unit visiting hours. I would sometimes be there from 9:00 AM to 10:00 PM without coming home.

Helping with just the day-to-day things. Helping with getting kids to and from activities, running errands, going to the grocery store, and helping with the laundry are just a few things that can really help.

Just being available. There are times as a patient, caregiver, or family member that we just need that shoulder to cry on or a listening ear. It can really go a long way to know that if you need someone, they are there to help you go through the good and bad times.

Sarah Ann adds...

By the time my dad's health had declined to where he was admitted into the hospital for longer stays, I was at the age where I had a boyfriend. He really helped us out a lot during that time period. It was a comfort to both of us to have someone who was there for me to confide in. He often gave me a ride to and from the hospital when we had bad weather, brought my mom and me food when we needed to eat (even though we often did not feel like eating). It helped my mom to know that I was safe and had someone helping me so she didn't have to worry about me and could concentrate on helping my dad. It helped me because he was the one person I wanted to be with when my dad wasn't doing well. I was very fortunate to have had a couple of boyfriends who were there for me through that time of my life and they were very considerate and helpful with the situation. I always looked at it as God put them in my life at the times he did to help me and be my support so I didn't feel so alone going through my dad's illness because I was a very quiet and private person.

Staying with the patient while his or her spouse or care provider takes a break, returns to work, runs errands, or attends church or temple will be deeply appreciated. Some families develop a schedule for this as well as a schedule for bringing meals to the patient and family at home. When bringing food, please keep in mind that many times the patient's food preferences will change drastically as a result of chemotherapy, radiation, and medications. Bruce found seasoned and spicy foods that he had previously loved became very hard to eat and digest. The comfort foods became standard fare.

Day-to-day tasks around the house and yard—laundry, lawn and/or garden care, snow or leaf removal, grocery shopping, and housekeeping—are also possible ways to provide much-needed assistance. Providing rides and assistance to and from medical appointments is also appreciated.

PART TEN

The Unspeakable That Must Be Spoken

How do I decide when it's time
to stop treatment?

What is hospice?

More...

98. How do I decide when it's time to stop treatment?

Mesothelioma is a disease that can be difficult to control. Treatments may work for a period of time and slow the growth of the cancer, but at some point the disease will come back or progress. Your doctor may have told you that your cancer can no longer be controlled or that they are no longer able to get ahead of the cancer because of its growth pattern. If this is the situation, you and your doctor may need to think about switching the focus of care to the control of your symptoms and make the decision to stop any other types of aggressive therapy. If your disease and its treatment are causing a significant amount of symptoms that are decreasing your quality of life, you may also choose not to take any further active cancer controlling treatment. It is not a sign of weakness to make the decision to forego further treatment. This is a personal decision and should be supported by all members of the family. There should be no contention at this time, but a coming together to assist the patient in living the best life possible under these difficult circumstances. This is a good time to do those things you've wanted to do but have been putting off for a later date. You and your family can make decisions about the future and get your financial and legal affairs in order. This is also a good time to talk with your doctor about the types of assistance or programs that are available to you and your family to help take care of your health care and other terminal needs.

99. What is hospice?

The goal of hospice care is to provide comfort to patients and their families during the last months of life. Hospice is able to provide support and guidance and ensure that all physical, emotional, and spiritual needs are addressed. The treatment focus now switches from control or cure of the disease to palliation and/or relief of symptoms, and the primary goal becomes trying to maintain the quality of your life rather than its length or quantity. If you decide that you do not want any more active treatment for your cancer or if your doctor tells you that your cancer can no longer be controlled, it may be time to consider hospice care. A large number of hospice programs have now been established throughout the country. Even smaller communities usually have hospice care available. To be eligible for hospice, your doctor must state that you are at the end stages of your cancer and have less than 6 months to live. This is a guideline they use because it is difficult to give an actual estimate of the amount of time a person has before death. To receive the best total care that hospice can provide a patient, it is best to utilize their services months before a person dies rather than in the last few weeks or days. Ask your doctor about hospice care and what is available in your area. The American Cancer Society is also a good resource and can give you detailed information about your local or regional hospice services.

Sarah adds...

Phil was a very independent and mentally strong man. The last 2 years of his life, his health started to deteriorate and we all could see that. Our decision to use hospice was primarily for Phil to have peace of mind that I would have some help and didn't have to do it alone. We had a wonderful nurse and hospice counselor who made themselves available to us for any needs we had. Again, we had a good understanding of the program and we communicated very well together about what we did and did not need.

Sarah Ann adds...

I remember very vividly when I found out my dad had signed with hospice. I was a sophomore in college and living in my sorority house. I had just made it back to my house from class when mom called me and told me that dad signed with hospice. That meant I had 2 weeks left with my dad before I was going to lose him for good. I hung up the phone and instantly started crying. I was standing in the living room and my house mom came over to console me. She hugged me for what felt like hours. I went home shortly after and spent the remaining time by my dad's side. We watched The Hangover *and* How to Lose a Guy in 10 Days *along with several other movies. To this day I still haven't been able to watch* How to Lose a Guy in 10 Days. *It was our movie and it doesn't seem right watching it without him. The hospice process was short and since he chose to stay at home and have a nurse come to him, it didn't really seem much different than our everyday life. Hospice is a huge step to take and you should think about it a lot before you make the decision. I also recommend that you talk with your family beforehand. I knew that it was going to happen and it made the blow a little easier to accept.*

Sarah adds...

Phil had made up his mind that when he was discharged from the hospital the last time that he would not be going back there to die. He asked Sarah Ann and me to let him die in his own home with just the three of us together. It was a hard decision because Sarah Ann and I knew that, due to his retaining CO_2 and the numerous times we had to put him on a ventilator, that we would know the symptoms to be watching for. Knowing that, we pretty much would know *the day he would die. It made it difficult to know we would be watching him take his last breath. We called our pastor to talk to us; we talked with our hospice nurse and decided it was the right decision for us. Phil and I had already made funeral arrangements and prepared as much as we could the prior year. It was important for Phil to take care of as many things as he could prior to his death thinking it would make things a little easier on Sarah Ann and me when the time came. Again, we sat and talked about this and decided that we would do it together and be there for each other on that day.*

Sarah Ann adds:

I didn't really do much planning when my dad was getting ready to pass away. The whole experience was surreal, and, no matter how many times I had thought about the scenario, when it came time to take action and prepare for his passing, I didn't know what to do. I did the only thing that made sense: I didn't leave my dad's side unless I had to. I was a magnet with him; I tried to soak up every last minute that I could. Emotions are at an all-time high when you know your time is almost out and even though it's extremely difficult to do, sit back, and, take a deep breath, try to spend the last few days laughing instead of crying or fighting.

Life After the Loss of a Loved One

Sarah says…

It has not been easy without Phil. I have good days and bad days and have accepted that as part of this journey we have all been on. Cancer brings a lot of things with it. The one thing the three of us held onto for 10 years was trusting God was in control of things and that we did not want to live with any regrets, and I can say that we have no regrets. We lived every one of those 10 years making the very best of them that we could. We felt from the beginning that our choices were to let mesothelioma take everything away from us or to fight with everything we had and make the best memories together and that would be what we fell back on to help us through these difficult days without Phil.

Sarah Ann adds...

Life without my dad has been anything but easy and I'm still adjusting and grieving. I have yet to fully come to terms with the fact that my dad isn't coming back. When he first passed away, I had a hard time caring about anything that went on around me. I didn't really go to my classes. The only thing I could focus on for about a year was that my dad was gone. It's been about 2 years since he has passed away and although I have picked back up with my normal life, I still find it very hard to date people because my dad will never get to know them, and every time I achieve one of my goals, it's bitter sweet because my dad isn't there to share it with me. I know he is watching over me. I will be reunited with him one day, but it's still not the same and doesn't take the sting away of missing him. Life never gets easier; you simply become more adapted, you learn to deal. And you become stronger. It's not easy and it never will be easy.

100. The battle is just beginning. Where can I go to get more information?

The next section lists some recommended resources for finding out more about mesothelioma.

Recommended Resources for Learning More About Mesothelioma

Media

21st Century Adult Cancer Sourcebook: Malignant Mesothelioma — Clinical Data for Patients, Families, and Physicians, by National Cancer Institute [eBook]

An Air That Kills: How the Asbestos Poisoning of Libby, Montana, Uncovered a National Scandal, by Andrew Schneider and David McCumber (New York, NY: Berkeley Books, 2004)

Dust to Dust, by Michael Brown (Arlington, TX: Michael Brown Productions, 2002) [DVD]

Outrageous Misconduct: The Asbestos Industry on Trial, by Paul Brodeur (New York, NY: Pantheon Books, 1985)

Organizations

American Cancer Society
The American Cancer Society has a number of publications on topics pertinent to mesothelioma patients and their families. The Hope Lodge provides free housing for patients who travel for treatment. Contact your local chapter or visit their Web site for a full listing of some wonderful resources.

Web site: www.cancer.org

Cleaning for a Reason
Cleaning for a Reason is a nonprofit foundation dedicated to providing assistance with house cleaning for cancer patients who need "one less thing to worry about." Based in Texas, this organization has a nationwide

network of individuals and companies who volunteer their cleaning services.

Web site: http://cleaningforareason.org

Phone: (877) 337-3348

Corporate Angel Network

Corporate Angel Network arranges free travel for cancer patients to treatment centers using empty seats on corporate jets. Eligibility is open to all cancer patients, who are ambulatory and not in need of medical support while traveling. Eligibility is not based on financial need, and patients may travel as often as necessary.

Web site: www.corpangelnetwork.org

Meso Foundation

The Meso Foundation offers hope and support to patients and families by educating them on the disease, helping them to obtain the most up-to-date information on treatment options, connecting with mesothelioma treatment specialists, providing them assistance, emotional support, and community with others.

Web site: www.curemeso.org

Phone: (877) 363-6376

National Coalition for Cancer Survivorship's Cancer Survival Toolbox

National Coalition for Cancer Survivorship has a free audio self-learning program to help develop some of the skills necessary to meet and understand the challenges associated with cancer.

Web site: www.canceradvocacy.org/toolbox/

Web Resources

CaringBridge

www.CaringBridge.org

CaringBridge is a free Internet service that helps families and friends keep in touch with loved ones battling serious illnesses. In addition to the updates, it includes a guest book where family and friends can return messages of support.

The Environmental Working Group

www.ewg.org

The Environmental Working Group's Web site has extensive information about the presence of asbestos in this country as well as information regarding legislative efforts, etc.

Meso Foundation

www.curemeso.org

National Cancer Institute's Malignant Mesothelioma Page

www.cancer.gov/cancertopics/types/
    malignantmesothelioma

National Cancer Institute's Mesothelioma Clinical Trials List

www.cancer.gov/search/ResultsClinicalTrials.aspx
    ?protocolsearchid=5639470

For the latest in clinical trials sponsored by the National Cancer Institute of the National Institutes of Health, you should use the above Web sites. The first one will take you to the National Cancer Institute's mesothelioma home page and the second will take you right to the mesothelioma trials.

Suggested Alternative and Complementary Medicines from Memorial Sloan Kettering Cancer Center

www.mskcc.org/cancer-care/integrative-medicine/
about-herbs-botanicals-other-products

A

Abdominal surgeon: A surgeon who specializes in surgery below the diaphragm.

Adjuvant chemotherapy: Treatment given after the primary treatment to increase the chances of a cure. Adjuvant therapy may include chemotherapy, radiation therapy, hormone therapy, or biological therapy.

Alternative therapy: Practices used instead of standard treatments, which are generally not recognized by the medical community as standard or conventional medical approaches. Alternative medicine includes dietary supplements, megadose vitamins, herbal preparations, special teas, acupuncture, massage therapy, magnet therapy, spiritual healing, and meditation.

Amphibole: A type of asbestos also known as brown or blue asbestos named for company that began mining it in South African. Exposure to this form of asbestos is known to cause mesothelioma, lung cancer, and other medical conditions.

Anemia: A condition in which the number of red blood cells is below normal.

Anorexia: An abnormal loss of the appetite for food. Anorexia can be caused by cancer, AIDS, a mental disorder (such as anorexia nervosa), or other diseases.

Anticipatory nausea and vomiting (ANV): ANV is nausea and/or vomiting that occur prior to the beginning of a new cycle of chemotherapy in response to conditioned stimuli such as the smells, sights, and sounds of the treatment room. ANV is a classically conditioned response that typically occurs after three or four prior chemotherapy treatments, following which the person experienced acute or delayed nausea and vomiting.

Arrhythmia: Any deviation from or disturbance of the normal heart rhythm.

Asbestos: A naturally occurring mineral composed of long thin fibers which, when inhaled or swallowed, are directly implicated in the development of mesothelioma, asbestosis, lung cancer, and medical conditions. It is a poor conductor of heat and does not conduct electricity and has been widely used as an insulator.

Asbestosis: A lung disease caused by exposure to asbestos. The lungs lose their natural elasticity, resulting in difficulty moving air into and out of the lungs.

Ascites (ah-SYE-teez): Abnormal build-up of fluid in the abdomen that may cause swelling. In late-stage cancer, tumor cells may be found in the fluid in the abdomen. Ascites is a common manifestation of peritoneal mesothelioma and can occur as a manifestation of recurrent mesothelioma after chest surgery for the disease.

B

Biomarker: A substance sometimes found in the blood, other body fluids, or tissues. A high level of biomarker may mean that a certain type of cancer is in the body. Examples of biomarkers include CA 125 (ovarian cancer), CA 15-3 (breast cancer), CEA (ovarian, lung, breast, pancreas, and gastrointestinal tract cancers), and PSA (prostate cancer). Also called tumor marker.

Biopsy: The removal of cells or tissues for examination under a microscope. When only a sample of tissue is removed, the procedure is called an incisional biopsy or core biopsy. When an entire lump or suspicious area is removed, the procedure is called an excisional biopsy. When a sample of tissue or fluid is removed with a needle, the procedure is called a needle biopsy or fine-needle aspiration. Pleural biopsies are used to make the diagnosis of mesothelioma.

Biphasic: A mesothelioma that has both epithelial and sarcomatoid elements. Also called a mixed mesothelioma.

Brigham and Women's Hospital Staging: Process developed at the Brigham and Women's Hospital to better define stage as it relates to surgery. It is meant to offer a better picture of what the expected outcome might be following chest surgery for mesothelioma.

Broncho-pleural fistula: A complication after extrapleural pneumonectomy in which there is a leakage of air from the closed bronchial tube.

C

Cachexia (ka-KEK-see-a): Loss of body weight and muscle mass, and weakness that may occur in patients with cancer, AIDS, or other chronic diseases. Cachexia is a common manifestation of late-stage mesothelioma.

Cancer center: A hospital that specializes only in the care of patients with cancer. A National Cancer Institute (NCI)-designated cancer center is specifically recognized and partially funded by the National Cancer Institute.

Cardiologist: A specialist in the treatment of conditions related to the heart that performs the appropriate tests to see if a patient is functionally able to tolerate surgery for mesothelioma.

Catheter: A tube that can be used to drain urine from the bladder; an intravenous catheter is used to give fluids in the vein.

Chemotherapy: Treatment with anti-cancer drugs. There are many varieties of these drugs that have different mechanisms for killing cancer cells.

Chest pain: Discomfort in the chest that can range from a feeling of heaviness to a constant boring pain that requires narcotics.

Clinical trial: A type of research study that uses volunteers to test new methods of screening, prevention, diagnosis, or treatment of a disease. The trial may be carried out in a clinic or other medical facility. Also called a clinical study.

Cobalt machine: A radioactive machine using a form of the metal cobalt, which is used as a source of radiation to treat cancer.

Complete response: The disappearance of all signs of cancer in response to treatment; also called a complete remission. This does not always mean the cancer has been cured.

Cough: The mechanism by which we clear irritants from the large breathing passages.

CT scan: A series of detailed pictures of areas inside the body, taken from different angles; the pictures are created by a computer linked to an X-ray machine. Also called computerized axial tomography, computed tomography, or computerized tomography.

Cytology: The study and categorization of cells using a microscope.

D

Debulking procedure: The removal of as much disease as possible with the goal of leaving only microscopic disease behind that is invisible to the naked eye.

Diagnosis: The process of identifying a disease by the signs and symptoms.

Diaphragm: The major muscle separating the abdomen from the chest. The diaphragm aids in our ability to take air into the lungs as well as expel air.

Due diligence: The level of judgment, care, prudence, determination, and activity that a person would reasonably be expected to do under particular circumstances. It is a medical term used to imply that a patient has investigated the many options available for him or her after a diagnosis is made either by using second opinions or advice from the literature or other experts in order to make a decision about how and by whom he or she would like to be treated.

Dyspnea: Difficult, painful breathing or shortness of breath; one of the early symptoms of mesothelioma in the pleura due to the accumulation of fluid in the chest.

E

Early mesothelioma: Mesothelioma discovered before the onset of major symptoms. For example, patients may be undergoing a routine procedure when mesothelioma is found without any suspicion of a malignancy, and usually the disease is limited to a single cavity with no evidence of distant spread or lymph node involvement.

Echocardiogram: A test that uses sound waves to create a moving picture of the heart. The picture is much more detailed than an X-ray image and involves no radiation exposure.

GLOSSARY

Empyema: Infected fluid (pus) in the chest that can result postoperatively as a complication of surgery for mesothelioma.

Environmental Protection Agency (EPA): The mission of the EPA is to protect human health and the environment. It is particularly concerned with the protection of humans against cancer-producing fibers like asbestos.

Epidural catheter: A catheter that allows injection of an anesthetic drug into the space between the wall of the spinal canal and the covering of the spinal cord. This is the most reliable means for short-term pain relief after an operation for mesothelioma.

Epithelial (ep-ih-THEE-lee-ul): Refers to the cells that line the internal and external surfaces of the body. Epithelial is also the term used to describe the appearance of the cells under the microscope for the most common type of mesothelioma.

Erionite: A naturally occurring mineral in the zeolite family of minerals with properties similar to asbestos. It is not currently regulated by the EPA.

Esophagitis: Inflammation of the esophagus, which is the tube that carries food from the mouth to the stomach. This most frequently occurs in the setting of chest radiation after an operation for mesothelioma.

External beam radiation: Radiation therapy that uses a machine to aim high-energy rays at the cancer; also called external radiation. Most commonly used after removal of an entire lung for mesothelioma.

Extrapleural pneumonectomy: Surgery to remove a diseased lung, part of the pericardium (membrane covering the heart), part of the diaphragm (muscle between the lungs and the abdomen), and part of the parietal pleura (membrane lining the chest). This type of surgery is used most often to treat malignant mesothelioma.

F

Fellow: A doctor who extends his or her medical training in a particular area of medicine such as surgery, medical oncology, and radiology.

Fibrosis: The growth of tissue containing or resembling fibers that can occur after radiation therapy or as scarring after any disruption of normal tissue.

First line: Refers to the first treatment you receive for your mesothelioma diagnosis. Alimta and cisplatin are the only first-line treatment approved in the United States for the treatment of malignant mesothelioma.

G

Gene therapy: Treatment that alters a gene. In studies of gene therapy for cancer, researchers are trying to improve the body's natural ability to fight the disease or to make the cancer cells more sensitive to other kinds of therapy by either adding a gene that was lost in the cancer or interfering with a gene that contributes to the growth of the cancer.

Genes: Inherited instructions or "building blocks" that determine our individual characteristics and control many processes in the body; genes are what make each of us unique. Genes play an important role in cancer and many therapies are aimed at manipulating genes.

H

Health maintenance organization (HMO): A form of health insurance combining a range of coverages in a group basis. A group of doctors and other medical professionals offer care through the HMO for a flat monthly rate with no deductibles. However, only visits to professionals within the HMO network are covered by the policy. All visits, prescriptions, and other care must be cleared by the HMO in order to be covered. A primary physician within the HMO handles referrals.

Heated perfusion: The delivery of heated chemotherapy chemicals to the chest and/or abdomen in the operating room after the majority of the tumor is removed.

Hemorrhage: In medicine, loss of blood from damaged blood vessels. A hemorrhage may be internal or external, and usually involves a lot of bleeding in a short time.

Hospice: A program that provides special care for people who are near the end of life and for their families, either at home, in freestanding facilities, or within hospitals.

I

Informed consent: A process in which a person learns key facts about a clinical trial including potential risks and benefits before deciding whether or not to participate in a study. Informed consent continues throughout the trial.

International Mesothelioma Interest Group (IMIG) Staging: A way of defining the size of the tumor and the locations in a uniform way that facilitates comparing groups of patients who undergo medical interventions. This is the most widely used staging system and is currently under review to be updated in the near future.

Intravenous: Within a blood vessel.

L

Latency period: The time between the actual exposure to a carcinogen like asbestos and the development of cancer, such as in mesothelioma.

Linear accelerator: A machine that creates high-energy radiation to treat cancer, using electricity to form a stream of fast-moving subatomic particles. Also called linear accelerator or a linac.

Local recurrence: Reappearance of the previously treated cancer at its original site; with mesothelioma, a local recurrence occurs in the pleura most frequently after surgery for the tumor.

Loculated: When fluid in the chest cavity or abdomen is unable to flow freely. We often used the term "walled off" to mean that the flow is interrupted by disease, scar tissue, or thick viscous fluid

Lung cancer: A cancer of the lungs that is comprised of different cells than those associated with mesothelioma. Lung cancer has many known causes including asbestos exposure. If you are a smoker and were exposed to asbestos, you have an increased risk of developing lung cancer more so than a non-asbestos—exposed smoker.

Lymph: Fluid composed of lymphocytes.

Lymph node: A rounded mass of lymphatic tissue that is surrounded by a capsule of connective tissue; also called a lymph gland. Lymph nodes filter lymph (lymphatic fluid) and they store lymphocytes (white blood cells). They are located along lymphatic vessels. The involvement of lymph glands by mesothelioma changes the stage to a higher one and is an indication of a more advanced tumor.

Lymphatic channels: Interconnecting tubes that link lymph nodes and allow flow of lymph.

M

Magnetic resonance imaging (MRI): A procedure in which radio waves and a powerful magnet linked to a computer are used to create detailed pictures of areas inside the body; also called nuclear magnetic resonance imaging. These pictures can show the difference between normal and diseased tissue. MRI makes better images of organs and soft tissue than other scanning techniques, such as CT or X-ray. MRI is especially useful for imaging the brain, spine, soft tissue of joints, and insides of bones.

Malignant seeding: Growth of a tumor at a site that may be outside its original domain because of contamination of a new site with malignant cells after a biopsy or from cells in a malignant effusion.

Mediastinoscopy (MEE-dee-a-stin-AHS-ko-pee): A procedure to view the organs and structures in the area between the lungs where lymph nodes reside. The tube is inserted through an incision above the breastbone. This procedure is usually performed to get a tissue sample from the lymph nodes on the right side of the chest.

Medical oncologist: A specially certified physician who treats cancer and delivers chemotherapy.

Mesothelial cells: A specialized layer of cells that form a thin layer along the cavity and internal organs. These cells are responsible for secretions that aid in cellular processes.

Mesothelin: A protein found on the outside of both normal and malignant cells. It is found in abundance in epithelial mesothelioma in addition to some other cancers. It can be measured in blood, urine, effusions, and ascites, and can aide in monitoring response to therapy.

Metastasis (meh-TAS-ta-sis): The spread of cancer from one part of the body to another. A tumor formed by cells that have spread is called a metastatic tumor or a metastasis. The metastatic tumor contains cells that are like those in the original (primary) tumor. The plural form of metastasis is metastases.

Metastatic recurrence: Return of the cancer at a site away from the original site.

Mixed: A description of cells found in a mesothelioma tumor sample. Mixed histology, also referred to as biphasic, contains both sarcomatoid and epithelial cells and accounts for approximately 20–35% of mesotheliomas.

Multimodality treatment: Therapy that combines more than one method of treatment.

N

Narcotic: An agent that causes insensibility or stupor; usually refers to opioids given to relieve pain.

Neo-adjuvant chemotherapy: Chemotherapy that is delivered before a planned surgical or radiation-based treatment.

Neuropathy: A problem in peripheral nerve function (any part of the nervous system except the brain and spinal cord) that causes pain, numbness, tingling, swelling, and muscle weakness in various parts of the body; also called peripheral neuropathy. Neuropathies may be caused by physical injury, infection, toxic substances, disease (such as cancer, diabetes, kidney failure, or malnutrition), or drugs such as anticancer drugs.

Nurse practitioner (NP): Registered nurses who are prepared through advanced education and clinical training to provide a wide range of preventive and acute healthcare services to individuals of all ages. NPs complete graduate-level education preparation that leads to a master's degree. They have prescriptive authority and work in collaboration with their physician colleagues.

O

Oncology: The study of cancer.

Occupational Safety and Health Administration (OSHA): A government agency that regulates the use of asbestos and sets the standards for its distribution.

P

Palliative care: Care directed toward the symptoms related to your cancer diagnosis. Palliative care is usually delivered by a team of trained professionals and can help with symptoms related to spiritual, physical, or emotional distress. The focus is not on your response to treatment but on your ability to carry out and enjoy your daily activities.

Paracentesis: Insertion of a thin needle or tube into the abdomen to remove fluid from the peritoneal cavity. Commonly used to make the diagnosis of peritoneal mesothelioma in patients with ascites or to diagnose recurrence of the disease in the belly.

Parietal pleura: The lining on the inside of the chest wall that is composed of mesothelial cells and is the target organ for asbestos-induced mesothelioma.

Partial response: A decrease in the size of a tumor or in the extent of cancer in the body in response to treatment.

Pathologist: A doctor who identifies diseases by studying cells and tissues under a microscope.

Performance status: A measure of how well a patient is able to perform ordinary tasks and carry out daily activities.

Pericardial effusion: A collection of fluid in the space between the heart and the sac-like protective tissue, the pericardium.

Pericardium: The heart sac that covers the heart.

Peritoneal mesothelioma: Mesothelioma that originates in the abdomen and/or pelvis.

Peritoneoscopy: The use of a laparoscope, a thick, lighted tube to examine the abdomen.

Peritoneum: The membrane the forms the lining of the abdominal cavity.

Phase I trial: A study to understand how a drug works and what dose is best tolerated in human subjects. Safety of drug dosing is the main goal of this particular phase.

Phase II trial: A study to determine if a particular drug is effective in your cancer and to monitor and record any side effects associated with the drug.

Phase III trial: A study to test the drug against the standard of care to see how it measures up in comparison.

Physician assistant (PA): A licensed professional who works under the supervision of a physician. They have prescriptive authority and work in a collaborative manner with their physician colleagues.

Platelet: A type of blood cell that helps prevent bleeding by causing blood clots to form; also called a thrombocyte.

Pleura: A thin layer of tissue covering the lungs and lining the interior wall of the chest cavity that protects and cushions the lungs. This tissue secretes a small amount of fluid that acts as a lubricant, allowing the lungs to move smoothly in the chest cavity while breathing.

Pleural effusion: An abnormal collection of fluid between the thin layers of tissue lining the lung and the wall of the chest cavity (pleura).

Pleural mesothelioma: Mesothelioma that originates in the chest cavity.

Pleural plaques: Areas of scar tissue on the pleura (lining tissue of lungs and chest). It is direct evidence of exposure to asbestos fiber.

Pleural space: The space enclosed by the pleura, which is a thin layer of tissue that covers the lungs and lines the interior wall of the chest cavity.

Pleurectomy/decortication: An operation for mesothelioma that removes the involved pleura and frees the underlying lung so that it can expand and fill the pleural cavity.

PleurX catheter: Refers to a tube that is inserted into the chest or abdomen allowing fluid to be drained in the comfort of your home. Patients and their caregivers are trained in how to drain these catheters, which has a low complication rate and is really quite simple.

Pneumonitis: An inflammatory infection that occurs in the lung.

Pneumothorax: Air within the chest cavity.

Positron emission tomography (PET) scan: A procedure in which a small amount of radioactive glucose (sugar) is injected into a vein and a scanner is used to make detailed, computerized pictures of areas inside the body where the glucose is used. Because cancer cells often use more glucose than normal cells, the pictures can be used to find cancer cells in the body.

Prognosis: The likely outcome or course of a disease; the chance of recovery or recurrence.

Progressive disease: Cancer that is increasing in scope or severity.

Protein: A molecule made up of amino acids that are needed for the body to function properly. Proteins are the basis of body structures, such as skin and hair, and of substances, such as enzymes, cytokines, and antibodies.

Protocol: An action plan for a clinical trial. The plan states what the study will do, and how and why it will do it. It explains how many people will be in it, who is eligible to participate, what study agents or other interventions they will be given, what tests they will receive and how often, and what information will be gathered.

Pulmonary embolism: Migration of a clot, usually from the legs, to the heart resulting in the blockage of arteries to the lung and resulting in acute shortness of breath. A possible cause of morbidity and mortality from operations for mesothelioma.

Pulmonary function test: A series of breathing maneuvers performed in a certified laboratory that measures the lung capacity and the force with which an individual can inhale and exhale.

Q

Quantitative lung perfusion scan: A radioactive nuclear scan that allows the measurement of the function of individual lung segments that can be used to determine how an individual will tolerate loss of lung function for an operation for mesothelioma.

R

Radiation: Energy released in the form of particles or electromagnetic waves. Common sources of radiation include radon gas, cosmic rays from outer space, and medical X-rays.

Radiation oncologist: A physician who delivers radiation.

Recurrence: The return of cancer after the tumor had disappeared at the same site as the original (primary) tumor or in another location.

Recurrent cancer: Cancer that has returned after a period of time during which the cancer could not be detected. The cancer may come back to the same site as the original (primary) tumor or to another place in the body.

Red blood cell: A cell that carries oxygen to all parts of the body; also called an erythrocyte.

Referral: A seeking out of expert consultation by a primary physician. The expert may or may not be associated with a cancer center.

Regional recurrence: Return of the cancer in a location close to the original cancer.

Research nurse: A nurse who is responsible for ensuring that a clinical trial is conducted according to standard regulated by the protocol sponsors and institutional review board.

Response: The results measured either by X-ray or physical exam of treatment that compares the status (usually the size) of the tumor before treatment to its status after treatment.

S

Sarcomatoid mesothelioma: The least common variant of mesothelioma, which has the appearance under the microscope of spindly cells that look like supportive or connective tissue.

Secondhand exposure: Exposure to asbestos that occurs indirectly, such as from someone else's clothing, as opposed to exposure in the working place.

Second-line therapy: Therapy that is introduced if a patient has failed to respond or is no longer tolerating the initial treatment.

Serpentine: A type of asbestos known as white or blue asbestos. The majority (95%) of the asbestos found in the US is of this type.

Simian virus 40 (SV40): A virus that has been associated with the development of mesothelioma. It is thought that the polio vaccine was contaminated with SV40 between the 1954 and 1963. Recent papers suggest that SV40 coupled with asbestos exposure increases the risk for the development of mesothelioma.

Stable disease: Cancer that is neither decreasing nor increasing in extent or severity.

Staging: Performing exams and tests to learn the extent of the cancer within the body, especially whether the disease has spread from the original site to other parts of the body. It is important to know the stage of the disease in order to plan the best treatment.

Standard of care: In medicine, treatment that experts agree is appropriate, accepted, and widely used. Health-care providers are obligated to provide patients with the standard of care. Also called standard therapy or best practice.

Supportive care: Care given to improve the quality of life of patients who have a serious or life-threatening disease; also called palliative care, comfort care, and symptom management. The goal of supportive care is to prevent or treat as early as possible the symptoms of the disease, side effects caused by treatment of the disease, and psychological, social, and spiritual problems related to the disease or its treatment.

Surgical oncologist: A surgeon who specializes in cancer surgery. This surgeon will perform your surgical biopsies and other operative procedures that you may require for your cancer.

T

Taconite: A rock that contains approximately 25% iron and as iron stores in the United States diminished, this rock became prized for its ability to extract iron from within the rock. This mineral is heavily mined in Minnesota, where an association with higher-than-expected cases of mesothelioma and asbestos-related diseases has been reported. Studies are underway to determine if taconite itself can be a causative factor in these diseases or if exposure to taconite increases the risk following exposure to asbestos.

Thoracentesis (thor-a-sen-TEE-sis): Removal of fluid from the pleural cavity through a needle inserted between the ribs.

Thoracic (thor-ASS-ik): Having to do with the chest.

Thoracic surgical oncologist: A board certified, general thoracic surgeon whose practice is almost exclusively the treatment of cancers in the chest .

Thoracoscopy: The use of a thin, lighted tube (called an endoscope) to examine the inside of the chest.

Tissue: A group of cells that gather together to perform a function. The skin is an example of connective tissue.

Toxic: Having to do with poison or something harmful to the body. Toxic substances usually cause unwanted side effects.

Tremolite: A type of asbestos which has contaminated the vermiculite mined in Libby, MT, and also has contaminated chrysotile (a serpentine asbestos) and talc.

V

Vermiculite: A naturally occurring mineral that is used for insulation. In Libby, MT, the vermiculite mine was contaminated with asbestos and many people have been exposed to asbestos and developed asbestos-related diseases due to this contamination.

Visceral pleura: The mesothelial lining on the surface of the lung that can also be a target organ for mesothelioma.

W

White blood cell (WBC): Refers to a blood cell that does not contain hemoglobin. White blood cells include lymphocytes, neutrophils, eosinophils, macrophages, and mast cells. These cells are made by bone marrow and help the body fight infection and other diseases.

Workup: A series of tests to discover information about the patient, most commonly to define extent of disease or suitability for a given treatment.